RECEIVE FREE INFORMATION TAILORED TO YOUR STAGE OF PREGNANCY

We believe that every mum-to-be should have access to trusted and practical pregnancy and parenting advice.

To receive your FREE checklist, specific to your stage of pregnancy and parenthood, simply scan the QR code below or visit the link and tell us if you're:

- Trying to Get Pregnant
- Just Discovered You're Pregnant
- About to Deliver Your Baby
- Already Given Birth

www.yourpregnancydoctor.com/bookpromo

As our way of saying 'Thank You' we'll also send you weekly information personalised to your specific stage of pregnancy.

YOUR PREGNANCY DOCTOR

The 50 questions you need answering

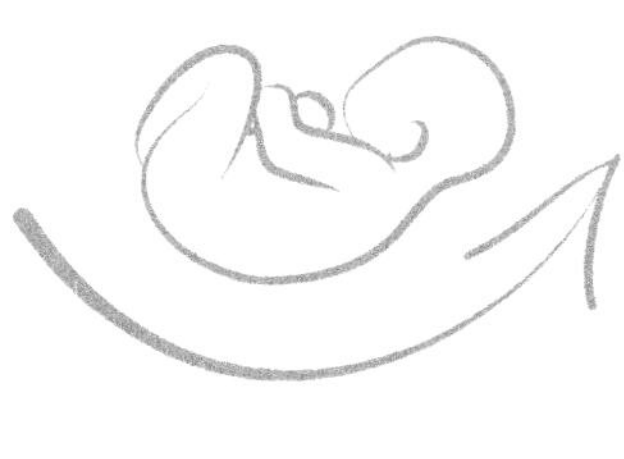

Dr. Keith Duncan

MBChB MD FRCOG

Your Pregnancy Doctor—The 50 questions you need answering

YourPregnancyDoctor.com

ISBN-13: 9781999986308

Interior design: Adina Cucicov

Limits of Liability and Disclaimer of Warranty
The author and publisher shall not be liable for your misuse of the enclosed material. This book is strictly for informational and educational purposes only.

Warning—Disclaimer
The purpose of this book is to educate and entertain. The author and/or publisher do not guarantee that anyone following these techniques, suggestions, tips, ideas, or strategies will become successful. The author and/or publisher shall have neither liability nor responsibility to anyone with respect to any loss or damage caused, or alleged to be caused, directly or indirectly by the information contained in this book.

Medical Disclaimer
The medical or health information in this book is provided as an information resource only, and is not to be used or relied on for any diagnostic or treatment purposes. This information is intended to be patient education, but does not create any patient-physician relationship, and should not be used as a substitute for professional diagnosis and treatment.

Printed in the United Kingdom, Canada and United States of America

TABLE OF CONTENTS

For more information sign up for our online video course Preparing for the Birth on YourPregnancyDoctor.com

YourPregnancyDoctor.com helps prepare you for life with your bump, your birth and beyond. Whether you're counting down to the big day, or you already have your baby in your arms you can get the information you need on our online video course Survival Guide to Life with Your Newborn.

FOREWORD

Pregnancy and childbirth can be a rollercoaster ride of soaring joy-filled highs and occasional crashing lows. Hormone-fuelled mothers and protective fathers are not always at their best and, particularly in the case of first-time parents, can be overflowing with questions.

Into this heady mix, Dr Keith Duncan MBChB MD FRCOG is a breath of fresh air—calm, kind, unfussy and experienced.

Over the last 25 years, he has delivered more than 3,000 babies in different hospitals across the UK. He works as a Consultant at Chelsea and Westminster Hospital in London and is the Director of the Chelsea Birth Clinic and a member of the British Maternal Fetal Medicine Society.

But despite all that, he remains utterly down to earth and accessible. As I discovered when I consulted him for the birth of both my sons, in 2011 and 2013.

Aged 43, during my first longed-for pregnancy, I was classed a 'geriatric' mother. After endless IVF and IUI attempts I was nervy (verging on the neurotic some—my husband included—might say) both about the pregnancies themselves and the births of my sons.

But somehow, with a combination of his gentle calm and northern charm (he was born in Blackpool and studied at Leeds University), Keith succeeded where my well-meaning husband had failed, making everything simple, straightforward and fuss-free.

As an expert in fetal medicine—with a special interest in high risk and multiple pregnancies—he performs all the ultrasounds himself, from five or six weeks to term, which provides a rare and comforting continuity, always taking the time to discuss the scans and patiently answer the myriad of my anxious questions.

He is exactly the doctor you want to be delivering your baby, whether for a natural, water, hypno or assisted birth, but particularly (as in my case) an elective Caesarean section.

Because as well as his lovely manner and impressive qualifications, his surgical skills, I had been assured by friends, were excellent. Endless delighted mothers commented on Mumsnet and raved about his calm professionalism.

They were right. After Keith's magic needlework, my physical recovery seemed faster than others in my antenatal class group, and my scar was quickly almost invisible.

I'm not sure anything can really prepare first time parents for the sterility of the operating theatre; the very medical atmosphere or, most of all, the imminent arrival of your first child.

But having experienced childbirth from both sides of the hospital trolley—he and his wife Sharon have a daughter Poppy—Keith knows just how strange, terrifying and wonderful it can be all at the same time and, somehow, helps his patients take the strangeness in their stride and embrace the joy.

He even managed to soothe my husband when a lovingly-prepared birth CD supposedly full of gentle jazz turned out to be completely blank—a more impressive feat, perhaps, than reassuring me during my epidural.

More tellingly, after thousands of births at every hour of the day and—more often than not—night, he still considers delivering babies the very best job in the world and experiences a surge of pure happiness at every new arrival.

This book provides a fantastically helpful and, as you would expect from its author, refreshingly straight-forward approach to pregnancy, birth and what to expect with your new baby.

For once there are no pointless frills or fluff—just really helpful and supportive advice on everything from early bleeding to whether you can safely dye your hair during pregnancy; varicose veins to guidance on how to decipher your own medical notes. Because after 25 years of experience, he knows the questions that new mothers want answering.

I couldn't recommend Keith, or this book, more. It will save a lot of new parents endless hours wasted Googling, and then worrying, unnecessarily—I only wish he had written it when I was pregnant.

~ Jane Fryer

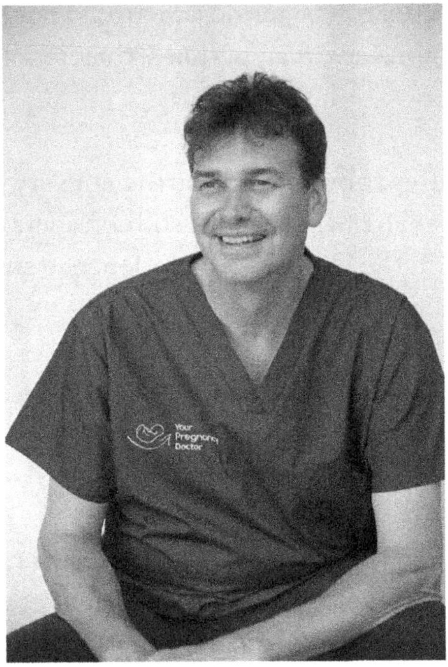

"I started Your Pregnancy Doctor to provide access to trusted pregnancy advice to every mum to be."

INTRODUCING DR KEITH DUNCAN

Dr Keith Duncan has been looking after pregnant women for over twenty-five years. He is a proud father to his little miracle Poppy, so has experienced pregnancy as a prospective father and birth partner as well as delivering over three thousand babies. He is a strong supporter of education, information and personal choice in childbirth, and in listening to the individual needs and wishes of each patient. Whether it's water births, Caesareans or hypno-birthing, his philosophy is to provide a positive birth experience for all parents to be.

Keith grew up in the North West of England. The son of a Scotsman, he was given a very Scottish name. Keith laughs that, to date, no one has named a baby he has delivered after him. He was named after Keith Richards of the Rolling Stones who were number one when he was born. He warned his mother he would do his best to emulate the rock and roll lifestyle, but ended up working a hundred hours a week as an obstetrician. He is proud of his Lancastrian roots and remains an ardent fan of Blackpool football club. He studied medicine at Leeds University and was inspired to become an obstetrician as a medical student when he was left in the delivery room with an expectant mother and ended up instinctively delivering her baby boy.

Dr Keith is currently a consultant at Chelsea and Westminster Hospital in London. He is Director of the Chelsea Birth Clinic and a member of the British Maternal and Fetal Medicine Society. He has served on the Council of the Royal College of Obstetricians and Gynaecologists, taking an active interest in women's health both at home and abroad. He has published a thesis on the assessment of development of the baby in the womb using magnetic resonance imaging.

An amateur genealogist, Dr Keith has delved into his own family history and discovered that his grandmother was orphaned when her mother died from bleeding in childbirth, sadly a common cause of death at the time. Wracked with remorse at what had happened to his wife, her father committed suicide. Their five children were placed in an orphanage and the family's property seized.

To Keith, this family tragedy is a sobering reminder of the risks of childbirth. It has inspired him to both appreciate how far obstetrics has come in the intervening years, and to personally ensure as many babies as possible enter the modern world safely and with their mothers in good health.

Dr Keith says:

Delivering babies is the best job in the world. At times, it can be unbelievably stressful, for the doctor as well as for the woman in labour. It is a job which demands long and unpredictable hours. My own family frequently has to take second place to ensure the safety of my newest arrivals. But in spite of these challenges, every time I deliver a baby and see that moment of pure joy when the family embraces their new member for the first time, I'm sure there can be no better feeling in the world. I know it's a job well done, and one I wouldn't swap for anything.

Dr Keith's story

I've delivered more than three thousand babies. They've come into the world head first, bottom first, as multiples and by Caesarean section. Each delivery is a unique experience as well as a privilege and an honour.

It's important to address the individual needs and wishes of each mother-to-be from first booking and throughout pregnancy and birth. Whether it's a water birth with hypnobirthing or an emergency Caesarean section, my aim is to provide a positive birth experience for all parents to be. The aim is to have a healthy mother bonding skin to skin with her baby and initiating breastfeeding with her partner or immediate family actively providing encouragement and support. This has been happening since the dawn of civilisation and is what separates us from other animals. In my opinion it's why we're the most successful species on the planet.

If you've ordered this book, you're probably either expecting a baby or you're planning for one, so let me be one of the first to say congratulations! Having a baby is an experience that's both intensely personal and universal to humanity. You can read about it and prepare for it, but there's no substitute for the life-altering experience of spending three-quarters of a year being pregnant and then delivering your baby.

My job as an obstetrician is to make giving birth as safe as possible. I am always alert, keeping an eye out for danger as I need to spot any warning signs early. Thanks to years of experience working under the guidance of eminent obstetricians and gynaecologists (and now with my own team), I've helped both mother and child avoid significant trauma and injury. But my role goes further than that—every birth should also be joyful. And each birth adds to my canon of knowledge, because every one is special and unique.

I had a fifty per cent placental abruption at week 37 which necessitated an emergency Caesarean section. Dr Duncan delivered his trademark brand of calm expertise and superior surgical skill with the speed and proficiency of a sniper, which saved our baby's life and prevented her from suffering life-limiting oxygen deprivation. He brought forward the operation on the theatre roster from a several hour wait to immediate. At the time of the operation the abruption, which had not presented dramatically, was already at fifty per cent and progressing. It is this instinct and expertise that I believe saved my baby from serious complications.

~ Jill, London

How I got into the business of delivering babies

The first baby I delivered as a medical student decided the course of my career. The moment he arrived in this world, I knew I was going to be an obstetrician.

Brought into the delivery room to assist the midwife, I was introduced to the expectant parents. The father, a well-known Leeds rugby league player, was a childhood hero of mine, so I was somewhat taken aback to see him out of his kit and in the delivery room.

The father sat in the corner, casually reading his newspaper, and seemed oblivious to the fact his wife was in well-established labour. As it was her fourth child, she was considerably more experienced in the delivery room than I was, and I thought absolutely nothing of it when the midwife popped out for a few minutes to talk to someone in the corridor.

But then she began to groan and roll her eyes and there was an overwhelming smell. I expected she had inadvertently opened her bowels, as is often the case during labour, and sprung forth to clean her up. I picked up a pad, pulled back the cover, and there was the baby's head, face down in a pile of poo!

I panicked and grabbed the baby to remove it—a normal reaction—and delivered the baby onto his mother's chest. At that moment, the midwife returned, saw the baby with their mother and screeched, 'What on earth have you done?'

Still in shock, I replied, 'I don't know!'

The midwife guided me as I delivered the placenta, and in those days, we stitched the mother too. My rugby league hero raised his head from his newspaper, asked, 'Is it a boy?' I told him that it was and then he rose and firmly shook my hand.

From that moment, I was hooked.

Since that day I've helped many thousands of babies into the world, but that didn't prepare me when it was time to see things from the other side of the hospital bed!

A doctor and a father

I met my wife Sharon relatively late on in my career, and it quickly became clear we were both keen to start a family. It took a long time for her to get pregnant, and just when we had decided to try for a baby via IVF, she fell pregnant. When I saw my daughter on the first scan, there was no better feeling in the world.

As a doctor, I am calm and reassuring, but like most expectant dads I had my anxieties. The problem was that I was too aware of potential pitfalls, so the pregnancy was difficult for me. I never rested, never relaxed. I scanned Sharon every Friday, and we sat there together, looking at the little one jumping around. I was a nervous wreck, checking that baby left, right and centre. So I understand what it's like to be a worried parent.

One of my fears was that as Sharon was a bit older, it increased the likelihood that the baby would have chromosome abnormalities. Like many parents, we thought long and hard about what tests to have, balancing the risks in our own personal circumstances. Every couple is different. Sharon and I decided not to have any diagnostic tests because we wanted a child, and would look after her, even if there were a possibility of Down's syndrome.

At the time of Poppy's birth, I didn't know whether she would have a chromosomal condition or not, but as soon as she emerged, it didn't matter.

Because she was covered in vernix caseosa (a natural white protective substance), I couldn't see her eyes, and so for the first half an hour I was convinced my beautiful baby didn't have eyeballs! That's how irrational even an obstetrician can be when faced with his own wife and child. My wife had a Caesarean section, and I can say with absolute certainty that the day of Poppy's birth was one of the best days of my life.

But this book is about you and your new baby. Over my years as an obstetrician, I've been asked hundreds of thousands of questions, both professionally in clinics and privately at parties. Some come up time and time again. I hope this book will answer those questions. There are also helpful tips and insights from patients and mums just like you.

For the sake of convenience, I'll speak to you as the mother. But this book is designed to be of equal interest to future fathers, family members and caregivers.

Pour a cup of tea, relax in a comfy chair, and join me in the pages ahead. Together, we'll strive to dodge the unpleasant aspects of pregnancy and childbirth whilst embracing the joy and fulfilment that can come only from becoming a mum.

Your Pregnancy Doctor

As an obstetrician, over my career I have had the opportunity to care for thousands of mothers and babies. But my practice is in Chelsea, in London, so I can only reach a tiny percentage of women.

Even though mums have been giving birth for thousands of years, it's still a tricky process. Globally, between a quarter of a million and 343,000 women are estimated to die each year from complications associated with pregnancy and childbirth. For every woman who dies in childbirth, around twenty more suffer injury, infection or disease, which means around ten million women each year are affected.

Infant and maternal mortality rates have steadily decreased in modern industrial societies. Today in the United Kingdom, the infant mortality rate is 4.2 per one thousand live births—but every infant death is a tragedy, and an important part of my job is to do what I can to make pregnancy and birth as safe as possible for both mother and child. That's why I started **Your Pregnancy Doctor**, to offer access to trusted and practical pregnancy advice to every mum-to-be.

YourPregnancyDoctor.com offers information written and checked by a team of experienced medical professionals as well as expert guidance, scientific research and sources of support to help each woman have a healthy pregnancy and a safe delivery.

Your Pregnancy Doctor supports mothers and families across the globe by providing a unique and consultant-led pregnancy platform. There is up-to-date, accurate and trusted information online and on video to help improve your personal pregnancy experience.

Your Pregnancy Doctor is committed to improving the lives and pregnancy experiences of millions of mothers and babies across the world by educating and empowering women and families. We want each individual to have a realistic understanding of pregnancy, bespoke to their own health and personal profile.

We are committed to increasing the accessibility of **Your Pregnancy Doctor** through technology, developing quality relationships and a dedication to excellent customer service.

Your Pregnancy Doctor provides trusted and valuable information, whenever and wherever you need it. **Pregnancy advice straight to your device.**

The Chelsea Birthing Method

I developed The Chelsea Birthing Method through my years of experience as an obstetrician (so named because most of my career has been based in Chelsea, in the heart of London). It is based on a simple assessment of each woman's individual risk factors and the likelihood of her achieving a normal birth without complications. It also factors in the chance of the newborn baby being admitted to special care or requiring antibiotics postnatally.

Don't panic. That doesn't mean pregnant women are assessed as machines rather than human beings. It simply means that each specific detail is scientifically considered. Afterwards, each individual's thoughts, wishes and feelings take priority. In my experience, it's much easier for someone to make choices when they're properly informed and they feel they are at the centre of their care, rather than part of some overarching paternalistic programme.

Most women want a normal, straightforward, vaginal birth. The good news is that over fifty per cent of the time they will achieve this. However, there are risk factors, including the age of the mother as well as their personal, medical and family history. By carefully considering all of these factors, I can give each woman a realistic statistical expectation as to their risk of a birth experience they don't want and what we should consider to obviate these risks. For example, this could include an elective Caesarean section for a mother whose first baby is lying in a breech presentation at term.

I also consider the use of the modern tools we have for assessment of the baby-to-be, notably ultrasound. I will identify the position of the baby, its weight and the location of the placenta. By considering the mother-to-be's health history and what the scans reveal, alongside their personal birth plan, based on my experience and published trials, I can indicate the risk of an emergency Caesarean section or instrumental delivery being necessary. I can also advise on the danger of any specific complications they might face.

The Chelsea Birth Clinic approach

Much like David Attenborough's presentation of stunning visuals on Life on Earth or Professor Brian Cox's metaphysical account of the world we live in, my approach involves a simplistic view of the risks and outcome of each individual's birth experience, something that has been a challenge since the movement of birth from home to hospital over the last fifty years.

This view may be challenged and criticised, but far too many women are not provided with a reasonable expectation of childbirth. In my experience, over fifty per cent of all women using the Chelsea Birthing method will obtain a straightforward, normal vaginal birth. Around twenty-five per cent will have either an elective or emergency Caesarean section and the remainder will have assistance with the birth, using instruments.

Each birth can be a positive experience, Caesareans and instrumental deliveries may not be listed in the birth plan, but they can still result in a beautiful healthy baby and a delivery both mum and partner can look back on with joy. Many potential parents have grave reservations about delivery with forceps or vacuum. It's understandable because they look rather like instruments of torture—but they are safe effective aids to delivery, when used correctly.

Among the vaginal births, there will inevitably be some who suffer damage to the muscles controlling the pelvic floor. This affects between three and five per cent of women and is more common in women who need instrumental deliveries.

In all groups, there is a risk of major blood loss (defined as more than 1.5 litres) but this is smallest in the straightforward vaginal birth and highest with an emergency Caesarean section when the baby is stuck low down in the pelvis, or in a complicated rotational instrumental birth.

At present, I do not have the tools available to accurately predict which group a first-time mum is going to fall in, which in the twenty-first century is disappointing. Historically, funding for research into labour has been notoriously difficult to secure. Therefore, much of the data is from databases which are often inaccurate.

One of the things that excites me about research is the potential to accurately assess women before, or in the early stages of labour. This would allow analysis and prediction of whether each woman is likely to be in the group who delivers vaginally without any problems, or would be likely to require an emergency Caesarean section. These are a group of women who seem to have a poorer birth experience.

Of course, it won't replace natural instincts, experience, professionalism and that all-important human touch, or what is traditionally described as 'bedside manner'. 'You can't please all people all of the time' is an often-exercised brief but I strive to do my best. My favourite writer Stephen King said, 'Talent is cheaper than table salt. What separates the talented individual from the successful one is a lot of hard work.'

Technology and medical advances can improve the process of labour and birth and ensure the safety and wellbeing of mother and baby. The Chelsea Method is about harnessing this, and empowering each woman to achieve the birth experience they imagined, whilst not feeling they have 'failed' if things don't go to plan. It also puts them in the best place to bond with their newborns as a family, with the closeness of skin-to-skin contact, as nature intended. The journey may be normal or complex, but there is a common goal for all of us, mums, families and caregivers.

THE FIRST TRIMESTER

"In the first trimester although you don't look pregnant your body is hard at work helping your baby grow and develop."

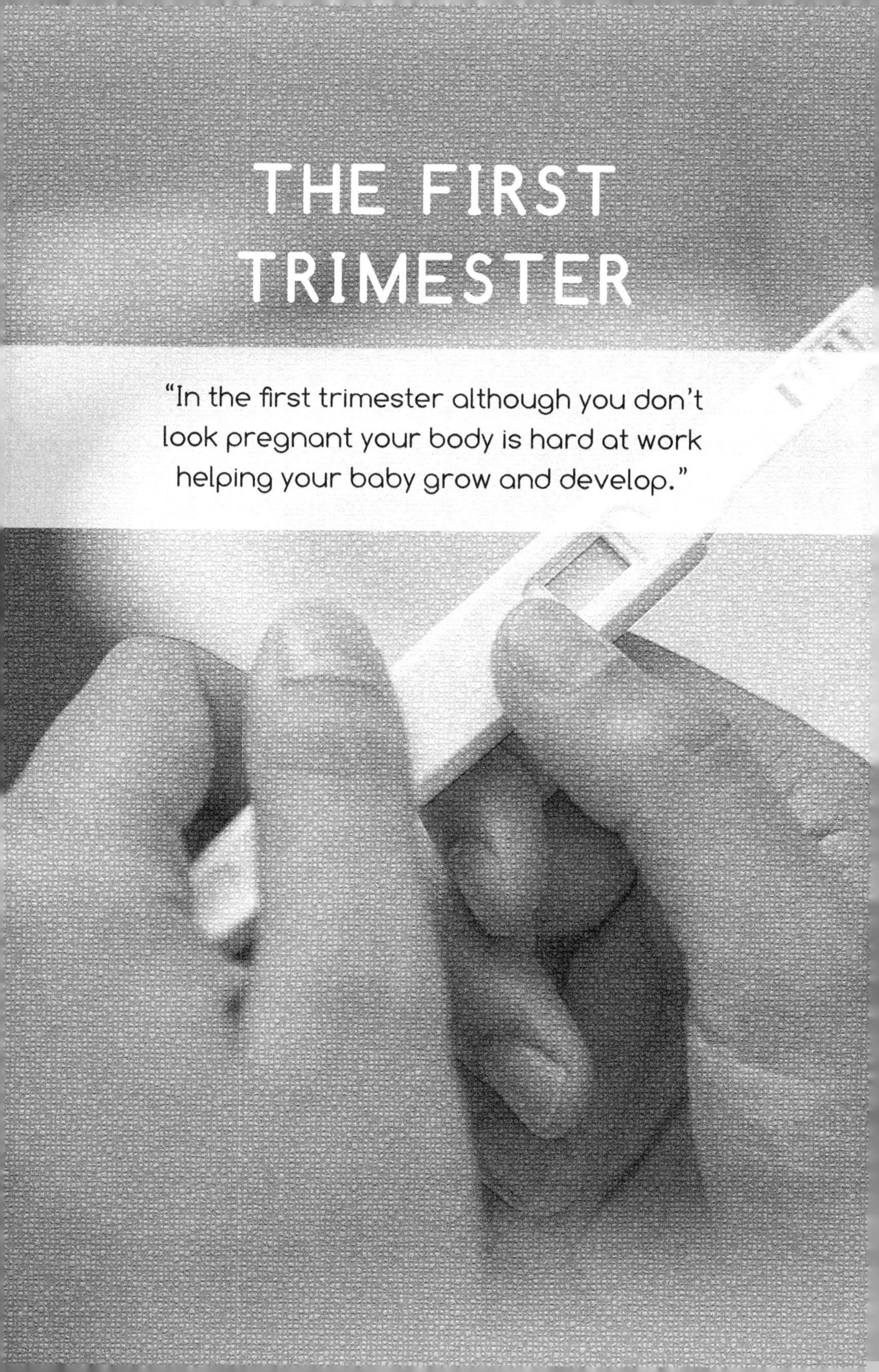

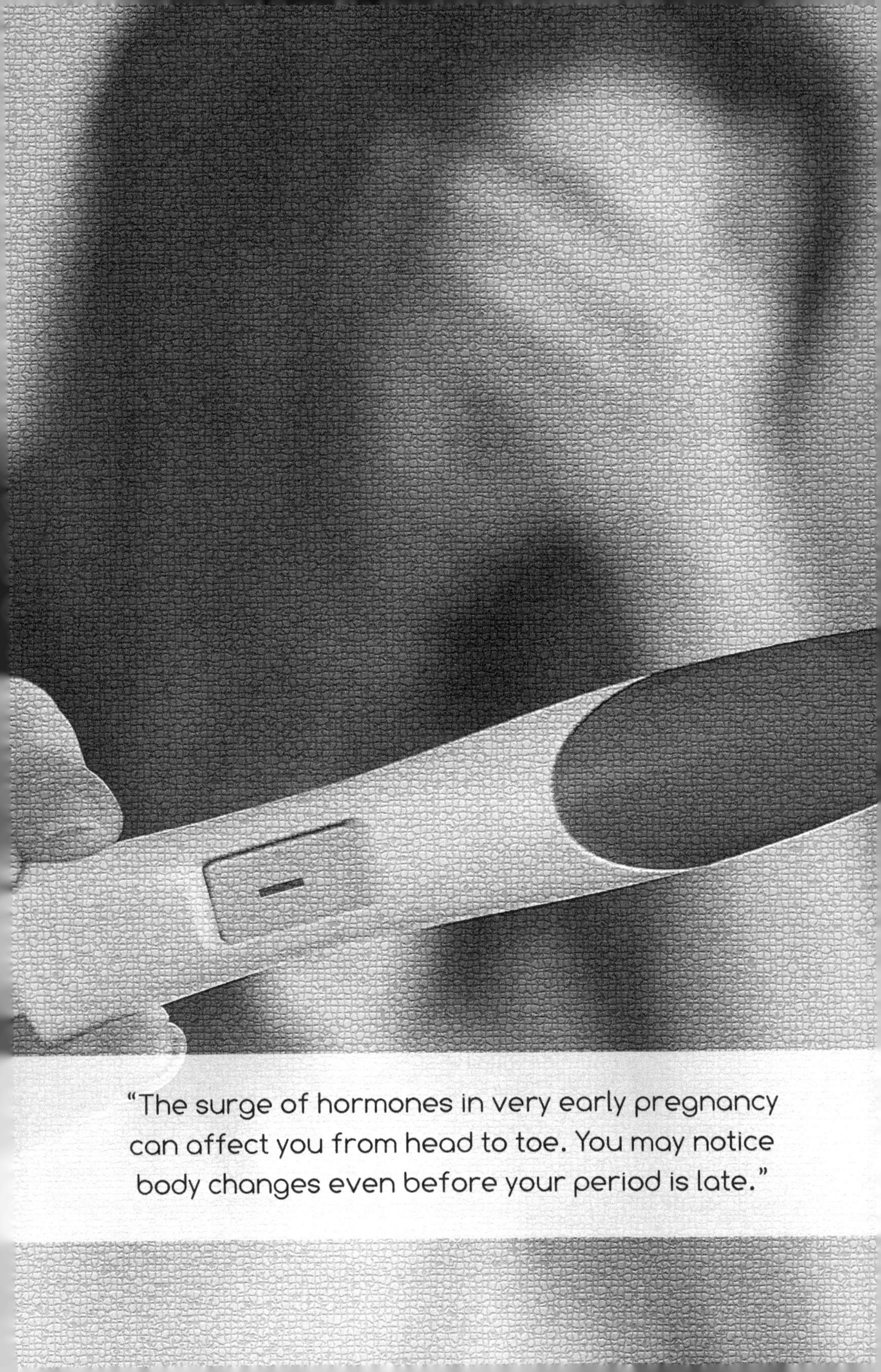

“The surge of hormones in very early pregnancy can affect you from head to toe. You may notice body changes even before your period is late.”

1

HOW CAN I TELL I'M PREGNANT?

You've done the deed and you're drumming your fingers impatiently and scrutinising your body to see if anything has changed. Even before the thin blue line appears on the pregnancy test, your body has already changed and is working hard to nurture the growing baby inside you.

There's a surge of hormones in early pregnancy that can affect you from head to toe. Although there's no bump to demonstrate your condition to the world, you may notice some body changes even before your period is late.

These are the top five early clues shared with me by the pregnant women I've cared for.

Tingly nipples

Pregnancy hormones boost the blood supply to your breasts making them feel prickly or tingly. This happens very early on, within a week of conception, and the sensation gradually passes as your body adapts to the hormonal surge.

Later, by around six weeks, you may find your breasts get more and more tender as well as becoming swollen and having more prominent veins. It's a little like they are before a period—but super-charged! Invest in a good bra to keep your breasts supported and comfortable.

Strange senses

Can't face your morning latte? Does your favourite perfume make you heave? The hormonal surge of pregnancy can have an early effect on your senses. You may go off certain flavours or find the scent of frying food in a restaurant makes you heave.

Pregnancy hormones can heighten your sense of smell, making it much more sensitive and meaning that aromas and flavours you used to adore can make you nauseous. One mum whose babies I delivered told me that the first way she knows she's pregnant is when the merest whiff of coffee turns her stomach.

A funny taste

My second pregnancy wasn't planned, although it was a lovely surprise. Our baby was around a year old and we had arranged for a romantic night away as a couple, with my parents caring for our little one. In the car, I commented to my husband that I had a funny taste in my mouth and if I didn't know better I'd think I was pregnant.

My period wasn't late, I felt totally well and frankly, with the lack of sleep, there hadn't been a whole load of chances to conceive! Anyway, I bought the test and boom the line was blue. I found out in the loos of the Ashmolean Library in Oxford. The rest of the day was a total blur. That funny metallic taste is a surefire early sign for me.

~ Jane, Leeds

An odd metallic taste in your mouth can be the first sign a baby is on their way. Again, pregnancy hormones are to blame, leaving you sipping water and brushing your teeth frantically to restore freshness.

That sicky feeling

Some lucky women don't suffer nausea and vomiting during pregnancy. However, for many, it can affect them day and night. Morning sickness usually appears at around six weeks but it can start as early as four weeks, especially in twin or multiple births.

A little blood

Sometimes when the fertilised egg attaches itself to the womb, the uterus lining bleeds a little. It's completely harmless and normal, affecting up to one in three women.

The confusing thing is that an implantation bleed happens at around the same time as you'd expect your period. The clues are that an implantation bleed tends to happen earlier, around ten days after conception. The bleeding is lighter with no clots, lasts only a day or so and tends to be pink or dark brown in colour.

Tiredness

Many women experience mind-numbing tiredness in the early months of pregnancy. It can be difficult to survive the day without grabbing a sneaky nap. The surge in progesterone levels may be the culprit. Much of your energy is being used to form the placenta, to increase the blood circulating and to build your new baby—is it any wonder you're exhausted?

Feeling faint

In pregnancy, your body works hard to increase the volume of blood, so your developing baby gets the nutrients they need. Your heart has to beat quicker to pump this extra blood around your body, and in the first few months, your blood pressure tends to drop. This can lead to dizziness, weakness and fainting. Stay safe by getting plenty of rest, standing up slowly to avoid dizzy spells and boosting your blood with iron-rich foods.

Urinary frequency

You'll need a urine sample for your pregnancy test as well as for every antenatal appointment—and in my experience, providing one shouldn't be a problem. Pregnant women seem to spend their lives on the loo. From as early as six weeks, you may start to wee more often. It's down to the hormones and the increased circulating blood, meaning your kidneys have to work overtime. It's totally normal but if you feel discomfort or burning, see your doctor because you may have an infection.

A late or missed period

This is the obvious one, especially if you're usually relatively regular. In fact, you may have a positive test before you notice any changes in your body. However, if your periods are erratic you may find that feeling sick, having sore boobs and spending all day traipsing back and forth to the loo are the first clues you're pregnant. If that's the case, congratulations!

The truth is that all the boob squishing and knicker checking in the world won't be as accurate as a positive pregnancy test. So why not get testing? I'll be crossing my fingers for you.

Pregnancy tests

Your mouth tastes funny, your boobs feel sore and you don't enjoy your morning cuppa. But are you pregnant or premenstrual? When you're trying to conceive, the time before your period can seem interminable, so how soon can you do a pregnancy test, how do they work and can you really trust the results?

What are they testing for?

Pregnancy tests detect the presence of the hormone human chorionic gonadotrophin (hCG) in your urine. It's produced by the cells that eventually go on to become the placenta. After the magical moment of conception, levels of hCG rise rapidly and some spills over into the urine so it's a pretty accurate indicator of who's pregnant and who's not

How early can I test?

HCG is produced as early as six days after fertilisation but it usually takes around two weeks for the levels to be high enough to reliably trigger a positive result. This is usually the time your period is due to appear, so when you're popping into to stock up on tampons you could invest in a pregnancy test as well!

Super-sensitive tests are also available. These are able to detect lower levels of hCG and can give a result as early as six days before your period is due. They may be described on the packaging as 'early' or 'first', and if you check the small print they should have a high sensitivity of 10mIU/ml compared to 40mIU/ml for the less sensitive tests.

How do I read the test?

The most important thing is to read the instructions, then read them again and follow them precisely. Brands can differ and they're not cheap, so it's good to get it right first time.

You'll need to get wee on the sensitive bit at the end of the stick. You can do this by collecting some urine in a pot or by taking the direct approach and holding it in the stream as you go to the loo.

That's the quick bit. The wait for the results to show can seem utterly endless, and if you peek too soon, you may not get the correct answer. Different brands show the result in different ways; there can be blue lines, pink lines, symbols or digital displays. There may also be a control window where you can check what a positive test should look like.

Are they accurate?

Modern home pregnancy tests are incredibly reliable and the good news is that if you've tested positive, you're almost certainly pregnant. If it's a negative though, there may still be hope. If your dates are wrong, you tested early, or your urine was dilute, it's worth waiting a while and testing again.

If you've recently suffered a miscarriage or had a termination it can take a little time for hCG levels to fall back to normal. Sometimes it's also possible to get a false positive result if you've been taking certain fertility medication or if the test is out of date.

Getting the right result

A negative test can be upsetting, so it's important to make sure the result is as accurate as possible. There are a few tricks to help you get the right result:

- Check early in the morning when the levels of the hormone will be highest.
- Don't drink loads of fluid before a test; it can dilute the hCG in your wee.
- Try to use the middle bit of the urine flow.
- Be patient. The earlier you test the more likely it is to be inaccurate. If you get a negative, dig deep, wait a few days and test again.

Where can I get a pregnancy test?

Pregnancy tests are widely available in supermarkets, chemists and online retailers. They can also be done free of charge at your GP's, sexual health clinic or local walk-in centre. Lots of women expect a test when they first see me or their GP. But be reassured, your tests are as good as the ones we have in the hospital or surgery.

"'Naegele's rule—add nine months and one week to the date of your last period."

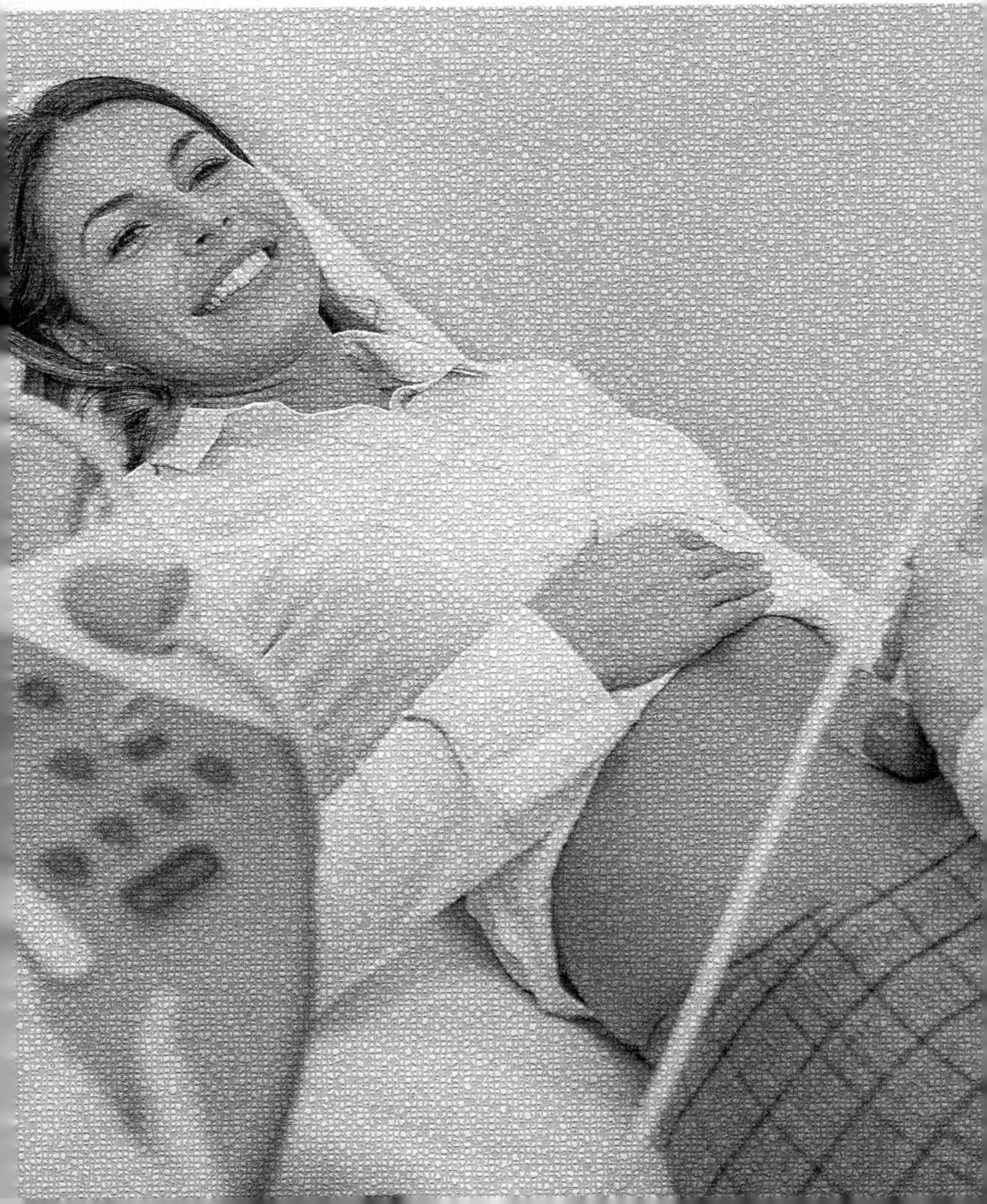

2

HOW CAN I WORK OUT MY DUE DATE?

The line is blue, you're officially pregnant and you're probably scrabbling for your diary and trying to work out your due date. It should be 40 weeks from the first day of your last period. Experience has taught me to rely on the dating scan for a more accurate idea, but if you're too impatient to wait until around twelve weeks, there are ways of working out when your baby is expected to make their entrance into the world.

Dr Keith confesses:

When it comes to due dates, I have to be honest and say that it's tricky to get the answer exactly right. Naegele's Rule can provide a useful guideline—you simply add on nine months and seven days from your last period to arrive at the due date. But research shows us that only a tiny five per cent of pregnancies actually arrive on their given date. So we're more likely to be wrong than right.

Dating details

From your period: Your baby's expected date of delivery is calculated from the first day of your last period. If you're organised and regular, and have it marked in your diary, you need to count 40 weeks on from that date. If you can't remember when your period was, try flicking through appointments, social events or meetings and see if that reminds you when you first came on.

From ovulation: Many of the women I see have been carefully tracking their ovulation prior to pregnancy. They may measure their temperature, use over-the-counter ovulation prediction kits, or watch their bodies for the tell-tale signs of ovulation. Check out the guide *Ovulation—the clues and calculations* or look at the following checklist for your body's normal timetable and the tell-tale signs:

Am I ovulating?

- If your cycle is regular, you'll probably ovulate 12 to 16 days before your period
- Your discharge will become watery, slippery and clearer
- Your body temperature will increase a little
- Hormones can be identified in your urine with predictor kits
- Some women feel abdominal pain or breast tenderness
- You may feel sexier and aroused

If you know when you ovulated, you'll have a pretty good idea when you conceived because an egg can only live for twenty-four hours after its release. Add on 38 weeks from the date of ovulation and that could be the day when you first meet your baby.

From conception: Sometimes there's only one date on which you could have got pregnant for the simple reason you only had sex once last month. That makes dating your pregnancy fairly clear-cut. Count 38 weeks on from the day when you did the deed and you'll find out your baby's likely due date.

Ovulation—the clues and calculations

Your body will change a little during your cycle. Some women notice breast tenderness, tummy ache, bloating or even a useful surge in libido when they ovulate. These symptoms are not the most reliable way of monitoring ovulation, but tracking these subtle changes may help you get in tune with your body and your cycle. If you want further confirmation, you can investigate further:

Do the maths

Didn't concentrate on your GCSEs? Don't panic. Ovulation calculations aren't complicated. The average cycle lasts between 23 and 35 days, with the first day of your period being Day One. The good news is that most of the variation tends to be during the phase before ovulation. The time after egg release is usually more consistent, lasting between 12 and 16 days. This means that if your cycle is regular, you are likely to ovulate 12-16 days before your period is due to appear.

Hot or cold?

Your body temperature changes slightly during the cycle. By tracking your temperature daily, you may notice a small jump in body temperature immediately after you ovulate. You can use a simple thermometer to measure at the same time each day. Don't make the mistake one of my patients made; it's fine to take the temperature orally rather than vaginally!

Testing, testing

The natural changes in your hormone levels can be reflected in your urine. Ovulation predictor kits can be bought over the counter to identify the hormonal surge that happens around the time of ovulation.

Mucous monitoring

If the mention of cervical mucus makes you go ewww, get over the ick factor because it can provide useful information about ovulation. It's natural. We're just talking about the discharge you've had constantly since puberty.

During much of your cycle, the mucous works to block the entrance to your womb and protect you against infection. However, as you get more fertile, your mucous should become more welcoming. Just before ovulation, discharge tends to be white or cream coloured, thick in consistency and slightly stretchy. When you're at your most fertile, your vagina becomes wet and more lubricated due to an increase in cervical mucous. It will also change in appearance, becoming thin, watery and transparent. I tell my patients that it looks a little like raw egg white.

Mum's conundrum

Can I work out when I conceived, and who the father is?

~ Anonymous, London

Dr Keith says:

This is a tricky one. You can definitely do some detective work if you can work out when you ovulated. It's usually fourteen days before your period arrives. But it's important to remember that sperm can be pretty persistent—they can usually live in the womb for three to four days, and sometimes up to a week. Anyone who you had unprotected sex with around the time of ovulation, and in the seven days before, could potentially be the father.

Your first ultrasound scan, the dating scan, may offer some more information. By careful measurement of your baby and assessment of the stage of development, your doctor or sonographer can calculate when your baby is likely to be born.

Mark your due date in your diary and carefully count back 38 weeks. That should give you a good idea of when your baby was conceived.

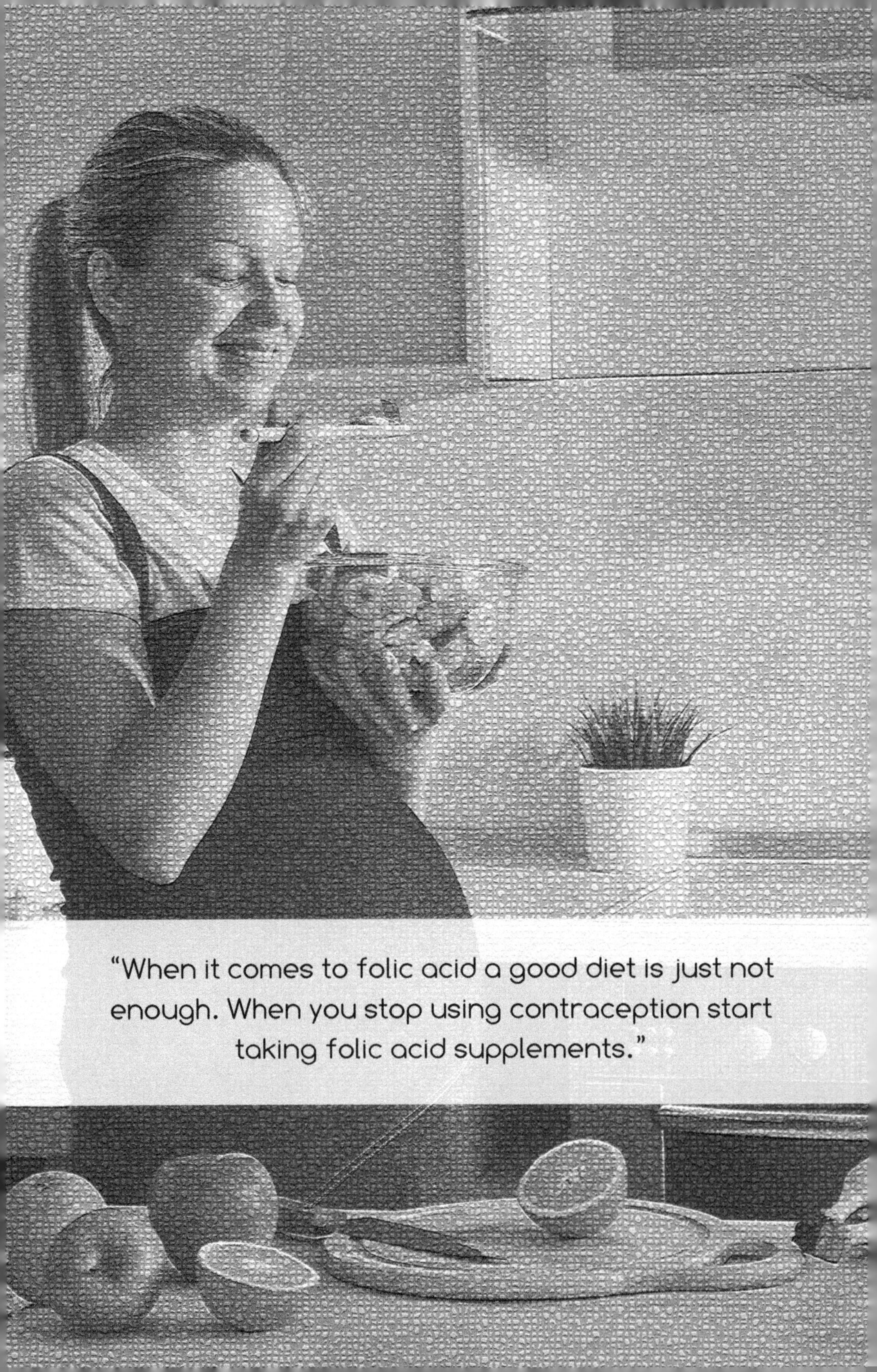
"When it comes to folic acid a good diet is just not enough. When you stop using contraception start taking folic acid supplements."

3

IS MY DIET GOOD ENOUGH FOR MY BABY?

From the first moment of fertilisation your body is nurturing and protecting your baby. A balanced diet is important to provide the vitamins and minerals needed to support this extraordinary process of growth and development. But lots of evidence suggests that often our diets alone may not provide everything needed to give your child the healthiest start in life.

I tell my patients that in an ideal world they'd be able to get the nutrients they need from the food they eat. But in early pregnancy, a woman's life is far from ideal. Morning sickness, tiredness and the conflicting demands of work and family life can conspire to make it difficult for mums to eat as well as they should.

A number of women I see come into pregnancy having spent periods of time dieting, taking the pill or suffering heavy periods. This means that many expectant mums are already lacking vital vitamins and minerals, even before facing the challenges of pregnancy.

Building a healthy baby

When it comes to vitamins and minerals, you really are eating for two. The body's need for micronutrients in pregnancy increases threefold, but the calorie requirement only goes up by a paltry 200 extra a day. It's important to choose nutrient-dense food but it's also important to take a regular supplement.

The folate factor

Folic acid is a vitamin that plays an essential role in the healthy development of your baby's brain and spinal cord. Taking a daily supplement around the time of conception will help protect your baby against spina bifida and other neural tube defects. It should be continued for the vital first twelve weeks of pregnancy when the baby's spine is developing. However, it's safe to keep going for the whole nine months.

Food and folate

When it comes to folic acid, a good diet is simply not enough. Your body needs much more folic acid during pregnancy and although it's found in lots of foods (including green leafy vegetables, wheat germ, yeast and eggs), it rapidly loses its strength during storage and cooking. So although it is sensible to choose folic-acid rich foods, the Department of Health recommends a 400-mcg folic acid tablet daily from the time you stop contraception until you're three months pregnant

> *When I stopped using contraception, I put my folic acid tablets in the same place as I kept my pills, next to my toothbrush. It meant I never forgot them.*
>
> **~ Louise, York**

If you're at increased risk

Some women may be at an increased risk of having a baby with a neural tube defect. This could be you if:

- You or your partner have a neural tube defect
- You've had a previous pregnancy with a neural tube defect
- You or your partner have a family history of neural tube defects
- You have diabetes
- You are taking regular anti-epileptic medication

A higher dose of folic acid can really make a difference and help protect your developing baby. See your doctor as soon as you start trying to conceive for advice and a prescription for 5mg of folic acid each day until you're 12 weeks pregnant. They may also recommend extra screening tests to pick up any problems or put your mind at rest during your pregnancy.

But it's not just folic acid that is important for healthy growth and development:

Vitamin D

Vitamin D is essential for your baby to use calcium and build healthy bones. Many people are deficient in vitamin D, so it's recommended that women in the UK take a daily dose of 10 micrograms when they are pregnant or breastfeeding.

Our bodies can make vitamin D in sunlight but dark skin, an indoor lifestyle, gloomy weather and careful sun protection can leave our levels dangerously low. Taking supplements can make you happier and healthier, can support your baby's growth during their first year of life and reduce their risk of developing rickets.

Even with a supplement it's a good idea to boost the vitamin D in your diet. For those who eat dairy produce, cheese, yoghurt and milk and eggs can boost vitamin D.

For vegans, vitamin D is found in fortified foods such as breakfast cereals and fortified fat spreads.

Iron

Lots of women become anaemic in pregnancy because there's more blood circulating and the work of supporting your growing baby puts extra demands on your body. You can be more at risk if you're a vegetarian or vegan because you miss out on iron-rich foods like beef, lamb and the dark meat in poultry.

Anaemia can cause tiredness, listlessness and sometimes fainting. It can also lead to shortness of breath and a pale complexion. A supplement can help, but it's sensible to eat an iron-rich diet throughout pregnancy, which may prevent problems arising.

Beat anaemia by choosing:

- Green leafy vegetables and watercress
- Dried fruits such as apricots
- Vitamin C, from citrus fruits or juices to help your body absorb more iron from your diet

Vitamin B12

Cyanocobalamin or vitamin B12 is critical in the manufacture of red blood cells. It also helps with the processing of folic acid and works to keep the nervous system healthy and release energy from food. You can find it in dairy produce like milk, yoghurt and cheese as well as in eggs.

Good sources for vegetarians and vegans include:

- Fortified breakfast cereals
- Fortified unsweetened soya 'milks'
- Yeast extracts such as Marmite

Calcium

Calcium helps your baby's teeth and bones grow strong. You'll find it in dairy produce like cheese and milk as well as in fish like sardines. If you're a vegan, you'll miss out on calcium from dairy produce. Boost your calcium by choosing:

- Dark green leafy vegetables
- Pulses and beans
- Fortified non-dairy 'milks', such as soya, rice, oat or almond milks
- Fortified bread and bread products
- Calcium-set tofu
- Sesame seeds
- Dried fruit like raisins, apricots and prunes

As well as these micronutrients, zinc is important to maintain growth in your developing baby, copper helps form the heart and blood vessels as well as the skeleton and nervous system, and magnesium works to build strong bones and teeth, regulates sugar levels and repairs body tissues. Vitamin E works hard to maintain healthy skin and blood vessels, vitamin C helps your body absorb iron and also maintains a healthy immune system and the rest of the B-group vitamins are essential for the formation of healthy red blood cells, to release energy from food, and to maintain a healthy nervous system.

Belt and braces

Every woman should take a daily supplement to provide folic acid and vitamin D. But if you're struggling to get the nutrition you need, a multivitamin designed for pregnant women can provide these as well as the other important vitamins and minerals that will keep you well and help you build a healthy baby.

> *I felt terrible in early pregnancy, I ate absolute rubbish because that was all I could keep down. I literally survived on plain bagels, white toast and ready salted crisps. I'd read all this stuff about nutrition and I wanted to scream. I felt terrible, but the idea of oily fish, salads and vegetables turned my stomach. I took a multivitamin every day, it made me feel a little less guilty and you know what? My baby was gorgeous and healthy.*
>
> **~ Philippa, Gloucester**

Remember that micronutrients are active substances and you can definitely have too much of a good thing. In particular, higher doses of vitamin A can harm a developing baby. Choose products designed for pregnant women, never double dose, and speak to your doctor or midwife if you have any questions or concerns.

4

WHAT IS MY RISK OF MISCARRIAGE?

Most of the women I care for worry about miscarriage, particularly in the early months of pregnancy. Sadly, miscarriage is common in the first twelve weeks. Whenever it happens, it can be a distressing experience. However, it's important to remember that you are still much more likely to have a healthy, uncomplicated pregnancy.

Miscarriage facts and figures

A miscarriage is the loss of a pregnancy in the first 23 weeks. It's tricky to know exactly how many miscarriages take place. The truth is that frequently a miscarriage can happen before the mum even realises she is pregnant. The estimated figure is that miscarriage happens in up to one in four recognised pregnancies, with the great majority happening in the first trimester before 12 weeks.

A late miscarriage is fortunately much less common, so there is good reason to relax a little after 12 weeks. After 24 weeks, the delivery of a baby who has died in the womb is no longer described as a miscarriage but is referred to as a stillbirth.

Facts and figures can't express the pain and the individual stories behind the losses. However, many couples tell me they want to know the statistics to help them understand their loss and start to look forward to the future:

- Twenty per cent of women go to hospital with bleeding in the first twenty weeks of pregnancy
- Miscarriage occurs in around 10-25% of pregnancies, although some may occur in the first five weeks, often before a woman knows she is pregnant—known as a 'chemical pregnancy'
- Eighty-five per cent of miscarriages happen in the first twelve weeks
- In the UK, 50,000 women are admitted with early pregnancy problems every year
- After a normal scan, 95% of those with bleeding will go on to have an uncomplicated pregnancy
- Over half of women with bleeding before 20 weeks will continue their pregnancy

Miscarriage risk

Some women do have a slightly higher risk of having a miscarriage. This includes those with underlying health problems and older mothers. Women who make potentially harmful lifestyle choices (such as heavy drinking of alcohol or caffeine, smoking and taking recreational drugs) can also be more likely to suffer pregnancy loss.

Although you cannot have any impact on chromosomal conditions or your age, there are some things you can do to bring down your overall risk of having a miscarriage. By getting to a healthy BMI, eating a balanced diet, kicking any bad habits and cutting down to 200mg of caffeine a day, you may help increase your chances of continuing your pregnancy and giving birth to a strong and healthy baby.

Early miscarriage

More than 85% of miscarriages happen in the first 12 weeks of pregnancy. These are known as 'early miscarriages'.

Causes of early miscarriage

It is thought that many pregnancies may be lost early, in the first five weeks, often before a mum knows she's expecting. The cause of many early miscarriages is not fully understood. However, it is believed that most are caused by chromosomal problems in the developing baby. Later, problems with the placenta can also lead to pregnancy loss.

Chromosomal abnormalities

It can help to think of the chromosomes as the building blocks of our genes. They contain the blueprint for developing every single cell in the body, with fifty per cent coming from the egg and fifty per cent from the sperm. If there's a serious problem when they combine at the time of conception, or during early development, this can mean that the baby is unable to live and there can be an early loss of the fetus.

Around half of early miscarriages may be caused by these kinds of genetic problems. But before you start to worry, it's important to understand that this usually doesn't mean you or your partner are carrying a chromosomal problem. It's often a new abnormality in the baby and most couples go on to have a healthy baby in the future.

Problems with the placenta

The placenta is your baby's life-support machine. It links your blood to your baby and is the source of food, fluid and oxygen. If there is a problem with the development or function of the placenta, it can cause miscarriage.

I have been pregnant twice. The first time I had a miscarriage around six weeks. I was considered high risk. I had a pulmonary embolism when I was twenty-five. The cause was the pill. Therefore, my specialist team decided to put me on blood thinners during my pregnancy, which I had to inject in my stomach. I was scared that the blood thinners would harm the baby. When I found out I was pregnant two months after the miscarriage I went to my specialist immediately and my pregnancy was fantastic. My daughter is nine now and healthy.

~ Patty, London

Dr Keith says:

Pulmonary embolisms are blood clots that reach the lungs and block blood flow, resulting in a heart attack or other serious medical problem. Some birth control pills are known to cause these blood clots. In addition, women who have had miscarriages are often given blood tests to check for genetic problems that may lead to blood clots.

These inherited clotting problems affect about one in ten people. The fear is that having one of these clotting problems may cause clots to form in the placenta, choking the delivery of oxygen and nutrients to a growing baby.

Research in the past suggested having a clotting disorder can lead to sticky blood and the risk of miscarriage, so doctors may prescribe a blood thinner to help prevent pregnancy loss and growth problems in the baby.

What will happen?

If you have had an early miscarriage, you may notice some bleeding or suffer lower abdominal pain and cramping. Sadly, you may notice no symptoms, and discover your loss on a routine ultrasound scan. This is known as a **missed miscarriage**.

With time, a full miscarriage will usually happen naturally. However, this can take days or sometimes weeks. Some women prefer if this process is speeded up, so they can put this difficult and stressful experience behind them and start to recover physically and emotionally. This can be done by the use of medical treatment or by a small operation.

Will it happen again?

> *I felt anxious throughout the pregnancy due to the previous miscarriage. I kept thinking this pregnancy would end in miscarriage also. Compared with the first pregnancy, when I assumed everything would go perfectly, from the minute I found out I was pregnant, I did not allow myself to think ahead or get excited in case things didn't go well.*
>
> **~ Pauline, London**

The good news is that whilst miscarriage is common, recurrent miscarriage is not. Only two per cent of pregnant women experience two pregnancy losses in a row, and only about one per cent have three consecutive pregnancy losses.

The technical definition for recurrent miscarriages or 'recurrent pregnancy loss' (RPL) requires three or more consecutive losses of recognised pregnancies before week 20, or the fifth month of pregnancy. Currently, it isn't clear whether early pregnancy losses diagnosed by sensitive pregnancy tests and not by ultrasound should be included in this definition. Most doctors believe it is reasonable to send tests and start treatment of RPL after two consecutive miscarriages.

The risk of recurrence depends on many factors, including the cause of the first miscarriage, the age of the mother, and any previous history of a live birth. However, it's important to remember that most women with RPL have a good chance of eventually having a successful pregnancy, whether or not a cause is discovered and treatment initiated.

Looking forward

Your body is designed to recover physically from the demands of a miscarriage. However, when a baby dies it can be difficult to cope with your emotions and adapt to the loss of the baby you planned and the future you'd imagined.

If the worst does happen and you lose your baby, it can be a lonely and frightening experience. You may have avoided telling people about your pregnancy, which can add to your sense of isolation. Please understand that you are not alone. Even if a problem shared isn't exactly halved, it can help to talk to others about your feelings and your fears. Talk to your healthcare team and share your emotions with your partner, your family or trusted friends.

Mid-trimester loss

Most miscarriages happen in the first trimester. However, as many as fifteen per cent of miscarriages occur later (between 15 and 24 weeks), so they are not as rare as people think. In my unit, every month we see a patient who is suffering a late loss—it's one of the most upsetting and challenging parts of my job.

The sad truth is that we often don't fully understand the reason for late miscarriage, but there are a number of causes and conditions that could potentially increase the risk. The good news is that with early diagnosis of these, we can make a difference and prevent problems occurring.

Causes of late miscarriage

- **Cervical insufficiency:** Problems with the neck of the womb can make it more likely to open up earlier in pregnancy. This weakness can be caused by surgery to the cervix, including treatment for abnormal or precancerous cells. It can also be due to birth trauma, or there may be an in-built tendency.

  If your healthcare team are aware of the risk, they can start treatment to prevent the cervix dilating too soon. An ultrasound scan can be done to assess the length of the cervix. If changes are noticed soon enough, there is research evidence that hormone therapy with progesterone pessaries can significantly decrease the risk of miscarriage. Also, a special stitch can be placed around the cervix earlier in pregnancy (known as **cervical cerclage**) to prevent premature dilatation.

- **Infection:** Infections can really take their toll on your body, and that's especially true in pregnancy. Any severe infection such as a UTI spreading to the kidneys, septicaemia or bad gastroenteritis (especially bacterial infections) can increase the risk of pregnancy loss.

  Pelvic and vaginal infections can be a particular problem. If they spread to the womb, they can make the membranes inflamed, a condition known as **chorioamnionitis**, which can kick off contractions and miscarriage. Although this is thankfully rare, it's essential to get medical help promptly if you are feverish and unwell or have an unpleasant or smelly discharge.

- **Illness:** When you have a chronic health condition, you become used to carefully managing your own health. This is particularly vital when you're expecting because chronic health conditions like diabetes, thyroid problems, high blood-pressure and kidney disease can increase the risk of miscarriage.

It can really help if you get expert medical assessment and support early in pregnancy, or ideally when you are trying to conceive. This can ensure you're in tip-top health so your body is in the best condition to build a healthy baby.

- **Medication and treatment:** It's important to be vigilant and get expert advice before taking any medications when you're pregnant. A number of drugs, herbal remedies and essential oils may trigger pregnancy loss. Check with your doctor, midwife, pharmacist or therapist before taking anything—that includes 'natural' and common over-the-counter treatments.

- **Problems with the womb:** Sometimes the shape of the womb can affect the attachment of the placenta or the healthy growth of the baby. This is uncommon, but can be caused by problems during development or by the growth of fibroids. If this has caused a miscarriage for you in the past, it may be worth consulting a gynaecologist to consider whether surgery could make a difference, before planning any further pregnancies.

- **Twin and multiple pregnancies:** The extra size and weight of multiple pregnancies can put extra pressure on the cervix, and trigger early changes to the neck of the womb and the danger of labour starting too soon. This increases the risk of premature deliveries and mid-trimester loss.

- **Genetic problems and fetal abnormalities:** Some late miscarriages are caused by a problem with the chromosomes in the baby or developmental abnormalities that are incompatible with life. Although it is not a consolation for the loss, it can be reassuring to know that most women go on to have successful pregnancies in the future. However, it is worth further investigation and genetic counselling if there is a strong family history of pregnancy loss.

Understanding and planning for the future

After a late miscarriage, you may be offered tests to help understand what has caused your loss. This can include a post-mortem examination or autopsy, which I understand is difficult to consider when you're still reeling from your loss. However, these investigations can help you discover why you lost your baby and whether preventative treatment will be able to help prevent any problems in future pregnancies.

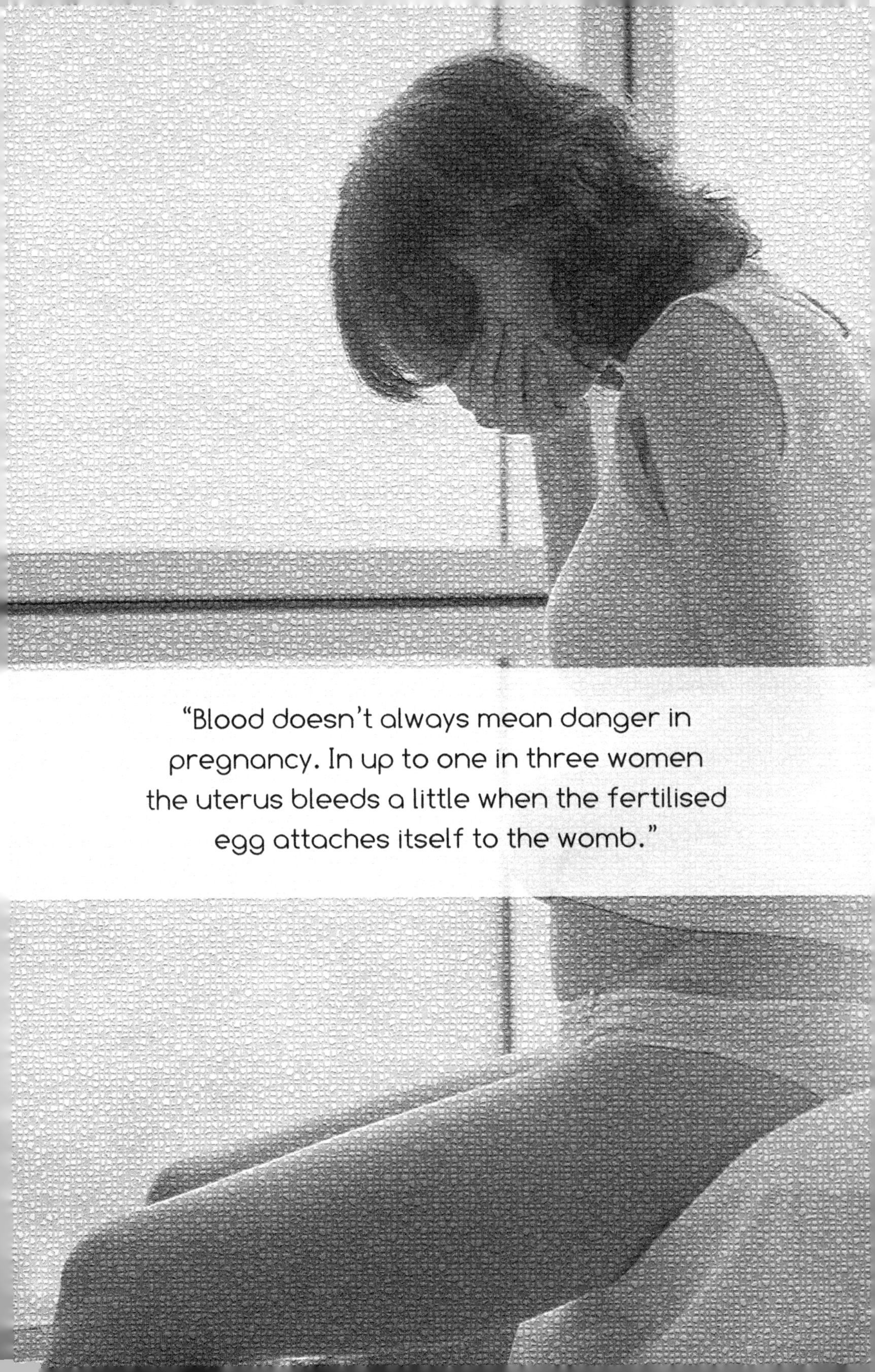

"Blood doesn't always mean danger in pregnancy. In up to one in three women the uterus bleeds a little when the fertilised egg attaches itself to the womb."

5

DOES BLEEDING IN EARLY PREGNANCY ALWAYS MEAN MISCARRIAGE?

To most women, bleeding in early pregnancy means one thing—miscarriage. It's natural to feel frightened but the Miscarriage Association says that around one in four women has some bleeding in the early stages of pregnancy and most go on to have a normal, healthy baby.

It's important to take any bleeding seriously, especially if you're in pain, but try not to assume the worst.

Implantation bleed

When you're trying to conceive and your period is promisingly late, the sight of blood in your pants or on the pad can be devastating. Don't despair though, it may be the first sign that changes are happening in your body. Sometimes when the fertilised egg attaches itself to the womb, the uterus lining bleeds a little. It's completely harmless and normal, affecting as many as a third of women.

The tricky thing is that an implantation bleed happens at pretty much the same time as you'd expect to menstruate. So is it pregnancy or your period? The clue is to inspect the blood and the level of flow. Don't worry, I'm not talking about a CSI-style analysis. A quick glance at the pad will give you a clue:

Colour: Implantation bleeding is often pink or light brown in colour, whereas your period blood may tend to be bright or dark red.

Go with the flow: Implantation bleeding is usually lighter than a period with no clots. Periods can start off light but the flow usually increases. If your bleeding hasn't got any heavier, it may be time to pee on a stick.

Patchy pattern: Menstrual flow is usually pretty steady and continuous throughout your period. Implantation bleeding tends to be more unpredictable and can come and go.

Short and sweet: When the fertilised egg implants in the womb you may get spotting for one or two days. Your period would normally last between four and seven days, so short is definitely sweet if you're trying to conceive.

Period pain? You probably know that your period can bring crampy lower abdominal pains along with it. You can get a little cramping when your baby first implants too. However, cramps from your period are much stronger and more intense.

If your bleeding is appearing on and off, if it's light and pinky-brown in colour and if your pain is a little less than normal, stock up on pregnancy tests. A new adventure may be about to begin.

Cervical bleeding

During pregnancy, the levels of the hormone oestrogen rise. This can alter the cervix, leading to a sensitive red area or erosion being exposed to the vagina. This area has a tendency to bleed, particularly after you make love. Fortunately, it's common and harmless and it usually settles down spontaneously after delivery. However, it is worth getting your doctor to check you over, especially if you haven't had a smear for a long time or you've had abnormal smear results in the past.

Ectopic pregnancy

An ectopic pregnancy is one that develops outside the womb. The fertilised egg may implant in one of your fallopian tubes or even in your abdominal cavity. As the pregnancy develops it can stretch the tube and make it rupture. This causes severe pain and cramping in your abdomen, which may be associated with pain in your back passage or spread to your shoulder blade.

There's often a little bleeding, but much of the blood can stay inside you, so you may only notice a small amount of blood from your vagina. This doesn't mean you're OK. An ectopic pregnancy is a serious condition that can put the life of a woman at risk. If there's a rupture, you can have heavy internal bleeding, so you may become faint and feel extremely unwell.

Fortunately, an ectopic pregnancy can be treated safely if picked up quickly. It's important, therefore, to seek medical help if you have pain or bleeding—even if it's only slight—in early pregnancy.

Many women in these circumstances ask whether it is ever possible to save the baby. I'm sad to say it's not. Surgery is needed to prevent rupture and serious risk to the mum. The operation is often done through a keyhole procedure or laparoscopy and sometimes through a cut in the abdomen.

The earlier the better is definitely true for ectopic pregnancies. If an ectopic pregnancy is picked up early on, it can often be removed via a small cut in the fallopian tube. If there has been rupture or significant damage, the whole tube may need to be removed. If this is the case, the other tube takes over and pregnancy can still occur naturally.

Miscarriage

Although I discussed miscarriage in the last section, I will go over it again for anyone who is flicking through and reading question-by-question.

A miscarriage is the term used to describe the loss of a pregnancy in the first 23 weeks. It can be not only distressing but also frightening and lonely. There may seem to be a host of different diagnoses and medical terms used by the professionals caring for you, and when you're confused and afraid it can be difficult to take information in.

> *I was ten weeks pregnant with triplets and running around at work when I started bleeding. I had no pain but the blood was pouring down my legs and I was terrified. To me, blood meant a miscarriage. I was hysterical as I drove to the clinic. I had a scan immediately which, thankfully, showed that the babies were fine. I had more bleeding a few weeks later but everything settled down and at thirty-two weeks I had three wonderful babies.*
>
> **~ Kimberley, Swansea**

Threatened miscarriage

A **threatened miscarriage** is said to happen if you have bleeding from your vagina when the neck of the womb is still closed. The bleeding may be light (like a period) or heavier with clots, and you may also feel crampy lower abdominal pain.

Bed rest used to be advised—but there's absolutely no evidence that this makes any difference to the outcome of the pregnancy. However, it's sensible to take things easy. You've been through a tough time, so be kind to yourself and don't overdo things. It's also a good idea to avoid sex until the twelfth week if you've had bleeding. There are hormones called prostaglandins in semen which can soften the cervix and start contractions, so it's safer to stay celibate—for the short term.

After a threatened miscarriage, your doctor will usually organise a scan or send you to an early pregnancy unit to confirm your pregnancy is still ongoing. If the scan result is normal, the chances are high—as much as 95%—that the pregnancy will continue without any further problems.

Inevitable miscarriage

A miscarriage is referred to as being inevitable if the neck of the womb is found to be open at this stage. When the cervix has opened, sadly nothing can be done to rescue the pregnancy.

An undiagnosed miscarriage

An undiagnosed miscarriage (sometimes still known by its old name of missed abortion) happens when the embryo dies in the womb but doesn't spontaneously miscarry. Women may notice a brownish blood stained discharge, or that the symptoms of pregnancy such as morning sickness or breast tenderness have subsided.

Blighted ovum

A blighted ovum is a pregnancy in which no embryo develops. The fertilised egg implants in the womb, develops a sac and the placenta continues to grow. The placenta produces hormones that give rise to the usual symptoms of pregnancy, such as sickness and breast tenderness, so it can be heart-breaking to find out that all is not well.

If there is bleeding, it is usually light, probably no more than a little brownish discharge at around 12 to 13 weeks. Sometimes a woman will have had no indication there is a problem until a later routine ultrasound reveals the devastating news that the baby hasn't developed.

What happens next?

If you receive the sad news that a miscarriage or a blighted ovum is confirmed, your doctor or nurse should support and guide you through how the loss of your pregnancy will be managed.

Often the pregnancy tissue will pass out naturally over the next couple of weeks. Sometimes you will be given medication to help this process, or you may prefer to choose a small operation to remove it if you would prefer not to wait.

The Rhesus factor

Women who are rhesus negative with rhesus positive partners need medical assistance after any episode of vaginal bleeding. Bleeding of this kind may sensitise the mother to form antibodies to her baby's blood, which can cause problems later in this pregnancy or in a future pregnancy. A treatment called *anti-D* can be given by your doctor to prevent these antibodies forming.

Pregnancy loss can be scary and deeply upsetting. Friends and family often don't know the right thing to say and can come up with irritating reassurances or bland platitudes. Be kind to yourself and to them.

6

WHEN DOES MORNING SICKNESS START?

Your period's late, the pink line is glowing on your pregnancy test and your breasts are sore and swollen, so why aren't you throwing up?

It could be that you're one of the lucky twenty per cent of women who sail through pregnancy without nausea. Or, perhaps more likely it's a little too early. Most women don't start feeling queasy until six weeks, a full fortnight after their period was meant to appear. Rarely, it can strike as early as four weeks, especially if you're expecting twins or more. But if you're in early pregnancy and feeling fabulous, make the most of it. Next week you may have your head down the loo.

What causes the ick factor and when?

- The hormonal surge of early pregnancy can alter your sense of taste and smell, so you may be sensitive to some aromas and have an unpleasant metallic taste in your mouth even before your period is due.

- From around six weeks the hormones start to slow down the speed at which your stomach empties, increasing the feeling of fullness and nausea.
- The eighth week is when levels of the hormones human chorionic gonadotropin (hCG) and oestrogen really start to soar. These sudden changes in hormone levels can affect the centres in your brain in the same way as motion sickness, which leaves you sprinting to the loo.
- Those pesky hormones also act to relax the sphincter between the stomach and the oesophagus. This can allow acid to travel back up your gullet, especially when you're in bed. The result is heartburn, discomfort and (yes, you guessed it) nausea.
- Pregnancy sickness should start to fade as you enter the second trimester and usually disappears by fourteen to sixteen weeks. But the queasy feeling could still strike a little later on, when the baby is growing and pushing up on your stomach.

Why me?

The nausea is believed to be the result of the hormonal changes of pregnancy. They can affect your sense of taste and smell, making you sensitive to some aromas and giving you an unpleasant metallic taste in your mouth. To compound this, the stomach tends to empty more slowly. The emotional upheaval and total exhaustion of early pregnancy can really aggravate the problem. Some people are more likely to suffer from morning sickness. It may happen to you if:

- You get motion sickness or migraines
- You get nausea or sickness in response to the birth control pill
- You had morning sickness in a previous pregnancy
- You're pregnant with twins or more

Coping with morning sickness

Most of us have seen films and TV programmes showing pregnant women racing to throw up into the toilet. Even so, the relentless reality of pregnancy sickness can come as a shock. The good news is that there's lots you can do to help yourself and soothe the sickness.

Eat little and often

Although the sight of food may make you heave, you may find eating a little will help calm your queasiness. But don't overdo it. Your stomach empties more slowly in pregnancy, so choose small regular snacks and meals. Try eating every two hours and pick bland food that may be easier to keep down.

Breakfast in bed

When I'm pregnant I never get up until my husband has brought me a cup of tea and a ginger biscuit in bed. It stops me feeling nauseous and sets me up for the day—I wish he'd continue once the baby's born!

~ Debbie, Harrogate

You may find it better to eat before you get up and get going. Encourage your partner to spoil you, or keep some crackers, biscuits, or protein-rich nuts by your bed for the perfect stomach settling snack.

Sips not drips

It's important to stay hydrated to feel better and stay healthy. You'll suffer headaches, weakness and more if you get dehydrated. You may even need to be admitted to hospital for medication and a drip. Take regular small sips of clear fluid or experiment with sports drinks, consommé, squash or ginger beer to see what stays down best.

A little acupressure

Acupressure wristbands were designed to help stop motion sickness. They're based on ancient Chinese medicine, which has been practiced for nearly two thousand years. There is a small plastic button on the bands which presses on a specific point on the inside of your wrist. It's meant to affect the flow of energy (qi) and reduce sickness. Many of my patients have found them helpful and they are recommended in the Royal College of Obstetrics and Gynaecology (RCOG) guidelines.

Beat the burn

Heartburn can make nausea in pregnancy much worse. Avoid coffee, cola, tea, chocolate and anything spicy, which can trigger indigestion. A glass of milk, some dry biscuits or crackers may settle your stomach. If you're struggling, try some over the counter antacids like Settlers, Rennies or Gaviscon. They're safe if used according to instructions. See your pharmacist or talk to your midwife for advice.

Go gingerly

Ginger has been used as a traditional remedy for nausea for centuries, so it's definitely stood the test of time. Try making fresh ginger tea by slicing the root into boiling water, or if that doesn't appeal, stick to something a little sweeter. Try keeping some ginger nuts or ginger cake close at hand to nibble when nausea strikes.

Mineral matters

Women with lower levels of zinc and other essential minerals, such as potassium and magnesium, may be more prone to pregnancy sickness. Try taking a multivitamin specially designed for pregnancy every day from the moment you stop contraception and start trying to conceive. However, it's important not to overdo the supplements. In my experience, multivitamins can sometimes increase the queasy feeling. I usually recommend a B complex supplement, which contains the essential folic acid, to go with the recommended vitamin D supplement.

Fresh and fruity

It may sound strange but some women find that smelling lemons can soothe that sicky feeling, so if you're suffering, scratch and sniff!

Rest and recharge

> *Mentally I felt fantastic! Physically, from months one to five I was nauseated 24/7 and throwing up a lot. My mother had told me she had the same experience, so I took it easy and didn't beat myself up about it. I was also very tired and went to bed early every day. This was also good to manage the nausea. Since I slept more, I didn't know I was so nauseated.*
>
> **~ Patty, London**

Everything is worse when you're exhausted. In the first trimester of pregnancy, your body works incredibly hard to help your unborn child grow and develop. Be kind to yourself. Schedule regular rests and naps into your day. It's not laziness; it's the best way of staying happy and healthy.

Get help

If you're finding it difficult to cope, you're losing weight, or you're struggling to keep fluids down, see your doctor for treatment and support. Anti-sickness drugs can be a help for many women, and sometimes you may need a short hospital admission for fluids and further treatment.

Dr Manjeet Shehmar who wrote the sickness guidelines for the RCOG said

Women with persistent nausea can often feel that there is a lack of understanding of their condition. They may be unable to eat healthily, have to take time off work and feel a sense of grief or loss for what they perceive to be a normal pregnancy. It is therefore vital that women with this condition are given the right information and support and are made aware of the therapeutic and alternative therapies available to help them cope.

Sickness can be serious. It's essential not to ignore recurrent vomiting that means you're unable to keep anything down. This severe form of pregnancy sickness is known as **hyperemesis gravidarum** (HG). It's a serious but rare condition affecting only 0.5 to two per cent of pregnant women. Women carrying multiples, with a family history of the condition, or HG during a previous pregnancy are at higher risk. It hit the headlines when Catherine, Duchess of Cambridge, was hospitalised with the condition.

Hyperemesis can be miserable. We're talking about non-stop vomiting, and nausea that's so debilitating it's dangerous. The severity of the vomiting can cause dehydration, weight loss, and a build-up of toxins in the blood or urine called ketosis.

Fortunately, even women who lose weight due to vomiting in early pregnancy tend to deliver healthy, normal size babies. However, if you are unable to keep fluids down or are not passing urine frequently see your GP who will check your urine for ketones—you may need to go into hospital for rehydration with a drip.

7

HOW CAN I COPE WITH FIRST TRIMESTER TIREDNESS?

From the moment your egg is fertilised by your partner's sperm, your body is already creating a new human being. It is an amazing process—but it can also be totally exhausting. I find that women expect to feel tired when they're carrying a big bump in the last trimester, but the bone-numbing fatigue of the first few months can be a shock.

The problem is that in the first trimester, you look normal. Many people don't know you're pregnant but it's difficult to survive the day without sneaking off for a nap. Although there's no bump to demonstrate your condition to the world, your body is already hard at work responding to your changing hormones.

Why am I so tired?

Experts believe that the surge in progesterone levels may cause sleepiness and the feeling of fatigue in early pregnancy. Your energy is also being used to form the placenta and to increase the blood circulating to provide your baby with essential nutrients. Your heart is beating quicker to pump the extra blood around your body, and although we often hear about the problems of high blood pressure in pregnancy, in the first few months the blood pressure tends to drop. This can cause dizziness and faintness and may add to your fatigue. With so much going on, is it any wonder you feel exhausted?

Fighting fatigue

- **Listen to your body:** There are no medals for struggling on when you're feeling weak and wobbly. Listen to your body and grab sleep when you can. One of the Your Pregnancy Doctor team told me that she used to put her head down on her desk between patients in the surgery. She was sensible; I'm a big fan of the power-nap. Pregnant women are fantastic at sleeping for short periods of time and waking up full of energy. Naps can help you recover from chronic sleep deprivation and decrease the release of stress chemicals into your system, so your body, your mind and your baby will be healthier after a siesta.

> *I simply couldn't get through a whole day at work. I hadn't told anyone I was pregnant so I used to disappear at lunchtime and have a snooze in the back of my car. Luckily, no one ever spotted me! After twenty-minutes sleep, I felt able to face an afternoon in the office.*
>
> **~ Rachel, Bristol**

If you already have children, catnap when they do, go to bed at the same time as them, or perhaps your partner will take them out, so you have time to put your feet up.

- **Eat regular meals and snacks.**

I was pregnant with triplets and I noticed the tiredness within a couple of weeks. I was working full time and found it difficult to rest, although I did lie on the floor of the office occasionally after lunch. Once someone came in and thought I'd fainted!

I used to go to bed at eight o'clock every night for the first few months and we really couldn't go out much because I was so tired.

I ate lots of bananas and had dried fruit with me at all times, especially apricots. I didn't eat cakes and biscuits because I really noticed they gave me a sugar slump afterwards.

I exercised gently at the gym and found that really helped make me feel more energetic-although I still had to go to bed at eight!

~ Kimberley, Swansea

You may feel that caffeine and chocolate give you an energy boost—but there is a dip afterwards. Instead, choose wholegrain complex carbohydrate foods such as porridge, bananas or oatcakes. These provide a steady release of energy and also stimulate the release of the body's 'happy hormone' serotonin.

- **Rearrange your working schedule:** I understand this may be tricky, but it could make the difference between working efficiently and having to take time off sick. You may find you feel better in the early morning but need to leave early in the afternoon. Alternatively, you may be able to take some work home at weekends in exchange for a lunchtime siesta. If you're still having difficulty coping, consider taking a few days annual leave and do a four-day week for a while.

- **Get out and about:** A short walk in the fresh air may temporarily perk you up. Although the idea may be unappealing if your fatigue is overwhelming, it's worth a try if a nap is out of the question.

- **Look forward:** As the fourth month approaches, the fatigue tends to disappear. This is the time when pregnant women are said to bloom, and as your bump starts to show you may feel a welcome burst of energy. If you are still feeling drained and debilitated, have a chat with your doctor; there are a number of conditions which can make you more tired in pregnancy.

When first trimester tiredness could be a problem

Some conditions in pregnancy can increase your fatigue and sap your energy. If your exhaustion is debilitating, you're feeling weak, breathless or unwell, see your doctor for a check-up.

Anaemia

I kept on waiting to bloom in pregnancy—but by five months I still felt absolutely terrible. It was the sort of tiredness I'd never experienced before, I was simply incapable of getting through a whole day at work—I could barely walk up the stairs.

I had blood tests at twenty weeks, which showed I was anaemic. I was so relieved. It was great to know there was something causing my tiredness; I wasn't being wimpy. The iron tablets gave me shocking indigestion and constipation—but it was worth it, By six months I felt like a human being again.

~ Sally, Newcastle

You've increased the amount of blood circulating and are supporting your growing baby. This puts extra demands on your body and can lead to anaemia. Anaemia may make you feel tired and listless and sometimes faint. It can also lead to breathlessness and your friends may comment that you look pale.

Your doctor can check your haemoglobin with a simple blood test, however it is normal for the haemoglobin level to drop a little as your blood volume increases, this is a process known as haemodilution. If it drops too far, iron tablets can help build up your levels. It is also sensible to eat an iron-rich diet throughout pregnancy, which may prevent problems arising.

Beat anaemia by choosing:

- Green leafy vegetables and watercress
- Red meat and dark meat from poultry
- Dried fruits such as apricots

Vitamin C (from citrus fruits or juices) will help your body absorb more iron from your diet.

Get a good night's sleep

When you're exhausted, you expect to fall asleep the moment your head hits the pillow—but it's not always easy to drop off. Whether your mind is buzzing with worries about the baby, or you need to get up every hour for a wee, it can be difficult to get the rest you need. I spoke to some of my friends and patients to discover their top tips for getting a good night's rest:

Fit for sleep

Take some gentle exercise during the day, like a short walk or swim. Physical activity will make it easier to unwind.

Cut out caffeine

Avoid stimulants like coffee, tea, cola and chocolate in the evening. Instead, try a warm milky drink or sip camomile tea to soothe you to sleep.

Herbal helper

A muslin bag filled with dried lavender may help you relax and fall asleep—and even if it doesn't work, your bedroom will smell wonderful.

Bedtime bath

> *When I couldn't sleep in pregnancy, I added a handful of Epsom salts to my bathwater. In fact, I still swear by them now, and Poppy's eleven! They're incredible; you can feel the tension ebbing away. Afterwards, my legs feel wobbly and I'm so relaxed I can doze off.*
>
> **~ Sharon, London**

Have a bath just before bedtime. Try adding a few drops of lavender oil to the water or a scoop of Epsom salts to soothe your muscles and aid relaxation.

Get appy

There are some fantastic apps available to help soothe you to sleep. I tried one a friend recommended and I was asleep within minutes, so I'm a big believer. Try *Sleep, Digipill or Sleep Well Hypnosis* to help you catch some ZZZZZs.

Get wee wise

The increased blood flooding through your system is making your kidneys work overtime, so frequent trips to the loo may be essential. Prevent too many middle-of-the-night toilet trips by avoiding drinks immediately before bedtime. It's also sensible to make sure your bladder is empty before you go to bed.

Relaxation exercises

Help yourself switch off from the stresses and strains of the day with relaxation exercises. Make yourself comfortable in bed, lying on your side. Breathe slowly and easily and focus on each body part in turn:

- Pull your shoulders down, stretching your neck
- Stop
- Relax and feel the new position

Work through your body, stretching and tensing each area before stopping and relaxing.

Finish with breathing, sighing out slowly ten times before relaxing and repeating. These exercises are brilliant for later in pregnancy and during labour too.

If you are still struggling, it is usually better to accept the situation and spend some time reading or having a bath until you feel sleepy. Fighting to go to sleep will add to the tension of the situation, making dozing off even more unlikely. If all else fails, it's back to daytime catnaps again—but don't overdo it. Sleeping for too long in the day may make your night-time insomnia worse.

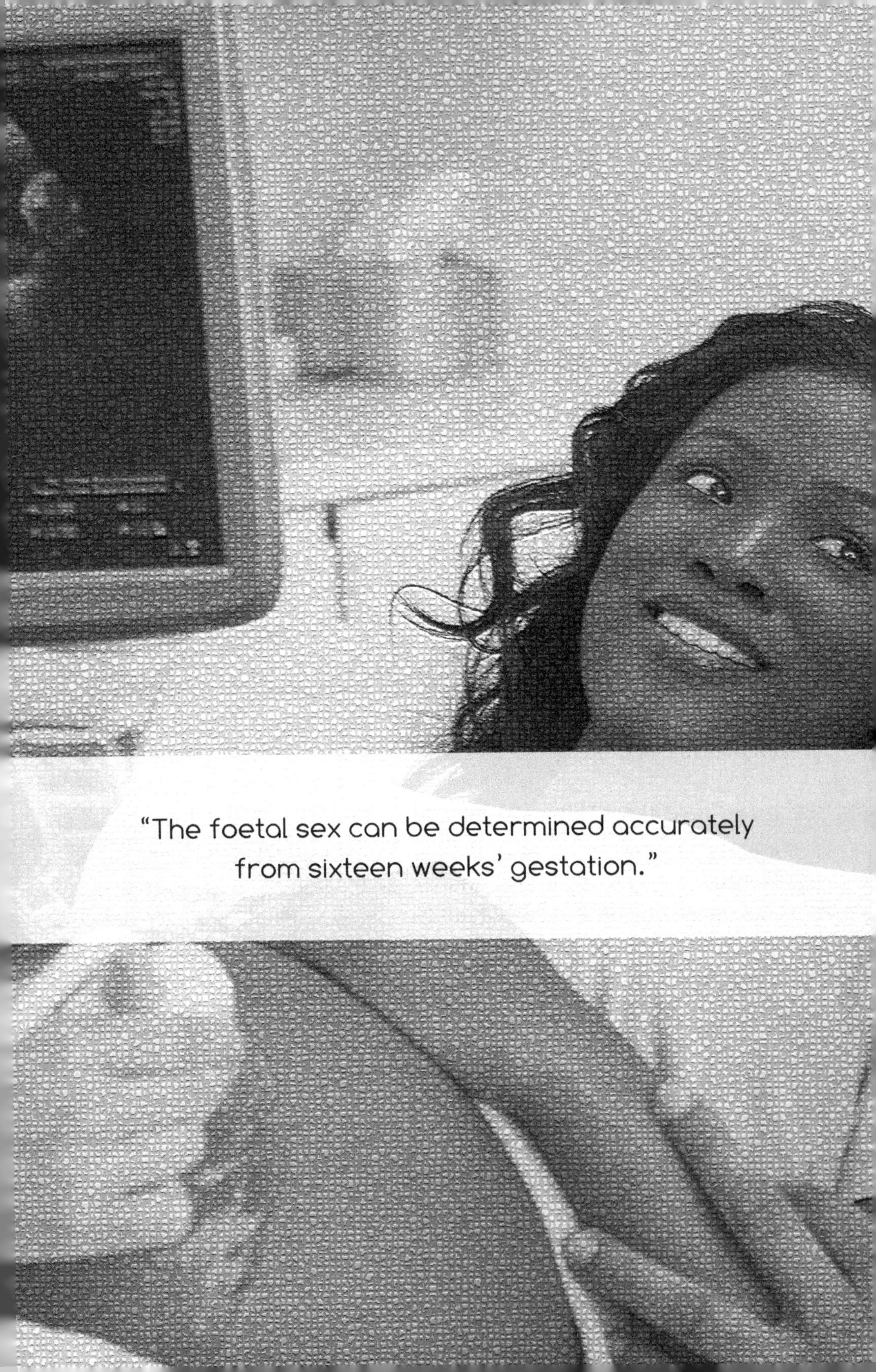

"The foetal sex can be determined accurately from sixteen weeks' gestation."

8

HOW SOON CAN A SCAN SHOW MY BABY'S SEX?

If you're itching to decorate the nursery in pink or blue and you simply can't wait until the mid-pregnancy anomaly scan, looking at skull shape or nub theory may be for you. It sounds like some obscure part of quantum physics, but it's actually a way of trying to predict your baby's sex by carefully examining the twelve-week dating scan.

What happens?

The dating scan is carried out between 8 and 14 weeks by a trained sonographer. You'll lie on a bed and move your clothing out of the way so the scanner can access your tummy, right down to your bikini line. A clear gel will be squeezed on your abdomen to improve contact between the ultrasound probe and your skin, so they may tuck a little tissue around your clothes to protect them and keep them clean.

The sonographer will press a smooth rounded device called a probe against your tummy. It sends out ultrasound waves and then collects them when they bounce back after reaching your baby.

These rebounding sound waves are translated into a moving black and white image of your baby on the machine. Don't worry if the sonographer keeps the screen facing them for much of the examination; it's really important they get a good view of the baby. They will make sure you get a proper look at your little one when the important checks and measures have been done.

A scan usually takes around twenty minutes. However, sometimes if the baby's in a tricky position, if your bladder isn't full, or if you've got high levels of body fat, it can take a little longer. Sometimes it may need to be repeated at another time. Not because there's a problem, but because your baby was a little shy.

What will it show?

At this stage, the sonographer will want to confirm all is progressing well with your pregnancy, check you're not having twins or more, and measure the baby so the estimated date of delivery (EDD) can be worked out.

A fold of fluid at the back of the neck called the nuchal fold may also be measured. This nuchal translucency (NT) scan is part of the combined screening test for Down's Syndrome.

The blobby, black and white pictures from an ultrasound scan are usually your first exciting glimpses of the baby growing inside you. The pictures may seem tricky to make out, but to a trained scanner they can reveal an enormous amount about your developing baby. You are usually able to get a printed picture to take home, which is where both skull shape analysis and nub theory comes in:

Skull shape

This theory is super-simple. If you're having a boy the skull will look larger with a square jaw. If you having a girl, the skull shape is rounder.

It could be true—in adulthood, men and women have different shaped skulls, with men's being heavier, thicker jawed and with a rounded profile and a sloping forehead. Women usually have more upright foreheads and rounder jaws. These facts are used extensively in forensics to identify the bones of men and women, so there is a sort of scientific basis for skull theory. However, the shape does change after puberty so it's not clear how big the difference will be between a little boy bean and a little girl bean. It's worth a good look at your scan to see though!

Getting to the nub of it

By twelve weeks your baby's chromosomal make-up is already set, and inside their bodies are already showing differences. If you're having a boy, his testes will have formed and will be pumping out testosterone, ready to drive the formation of the penis later in pregnancy. If you're having a girl, her ovaries will be developing ready to carry the eggs that will enable her to become a mum too, one day.

On the outside, things aren't as clear cut. Their genitals are really little 'nubs' known as *genital tubercules*. To be honest, the nubs look pretty similar in boys and girls, just little protrusions. Their developing genitals look a little like Ken and Barbie's smooth bumps at this early stage. However, experts in nub theory believe that the position of the nub (the angle of the dangle, so-to-speak) can provide a clue as to whether you're carrying a girl or a boy.

Up or down

Nub watchers tell me that if you're expecting a girl, the tubercule will stick directly outwards at right angles to the body. If the baby's a boy, it'll point upwards towards the head (feel free to insert your own joke here).

At this stage, your little one is a petite 6 cm and about the size of a Victoria plum, so the tubercule will be tiny. There'll have to be a fantastic screen image to properly capture the nub clearly, so you're able to make an assessment of the way it's pointing.

Does it work?

The sonographer at the dating scan for my second baby had a little look at the nub and predicted we were having a little boy. I was surprised because I felt the same as I had with my daughter a year or so before, but we were pretty relaxed about having a boy or a girl. At the anomaly scan, they firmly kept their legs closed, so we didn't know until our lovely daughter arrived several months later. I'm glad I didn't go mad buying boy's clothes!

~ Jane, Leeds

Dr Keith confesses:

I think there's some truth behind nub theory. In my experience, we can predict correctly nine times out of ten. The only problem is that people can get annoyed if it subsequently changes!

Lots of mums tell me they firmly believe that nub theory predicted the sex of their baby. The truth is that there's no real scientific evidence to back it up or disprove it. So feel free to examine those blurry black and white images with a magnifying glass—but don't sell the family silver to decorate the nursery in pink or blue.

9

WHICH FOODS ARE UNSAFE IN PREGNANCY?

In pregnancy, a healthy balanced diet will help maintain your wellbeing and provide your baby with the nutrients they need to grow and develop, but there are some foods you should stay well away from because they can put you at risk of food poisoning and may damage your unborn child.

Cheese

Cheese is a great source of protein and calcium but some cheeses can cause an infection called *listeriosis*, which could endanger your baby. Avoid mould ripened soft cheese, blue cheese and cheeses made with unpasteurised milk. That doesn't mean you have to ditch all cheese for the whole nine months. Try to pick hard cheeses like parmesan and cheddar for your cheesy fix. Avoid:

- **Mould-ripened soft cheeses** like brie and camembert
- **Soft blue cheese** like Danish blue, Gorgonzola and Roquefort
- **Unpasteurised soft cheeses** including goats' cheese

All about listeria

Listeriosis is an infection that can develop after eating food that contains the listeria bacteria. It's usually a mild illness lasting up to three days. Those affected have a fever, sickness and diarrhoea. These symptoms usually pass within three days with no need for treatment.

Some groups are more vulnerable to listeriosis including the very young, old and those who are unwell, frail or with weakened immune systems. Pregnant women are also at risk. If you're pregnant and show signs of listeriosis, it's important to see a doctor. You'll be given antibiotics to stop the infection spreading to your baby, and you may be offered extra ultrasound scans to monitor your baby's health and wellbeing.

Listeria bacteria have been found in pâté, soft mould-ripened cheeses, soft blue cheese, cooked sliced meats and some smoked salmon, although most supermarket brands are thought to be safe. The bacteria can be passed on through dirty nappies or stools from affected people or animals, so careful hygiene and handwashing is essential.

Raw eggs

Some raw or runny eggs can put you at risk of salmonella, a type of bacterial food poisoning. Eggs with the British Lion stamp have a low risk of salmonella, so should be chosen if possible. Supermarket ice-creams, mayonnaise and dressings are usually safe.

- **Make sure eggs are cooked through and be careful with foods like soufflés, mousses and home-made ice-creams and mayonnaise**
- **Choose eggs stamped with the British Lion to prevent salmonella**

Unpasteurised milk

Remember to stay away from unpasteurised or green top milk, whether it's from cows, sheep or goats—it can harbour listeria bacteria, so swap it for safe, pasteurised alternatives.

- **Do not drink raw milks of any type and avoid cheeses containing them**

Pâté

Pate can harbour listeria bacteria, whether it is made from fish, vegetables or meat

- **Avoid pâté**

Raw and undercooked meat

The good news is that most meat is safe to eat throughout pregnancy. However, it's important to ensure it's piping hot and cooked through, with no sign of pinkness or blood.

- **Cook meat and poultry carefully so it is not pink**
- **Be careful when barbecuing and defrosting meat**

Liver

You should also stay away from any type of liver because it's rich in vitamin A, which can be harmful to the developing baby.

- **Avoid liver**
- **Avoid liver products such as pâté and liver sausage**

Cured and continental meats

Cured meats like Parma ham or salami have not been cooked and may carry a small risk of listeriosis. It's sensible to avoid them in pregnancy.

- **Take care with products like salami and chorizo as well as Serrano and Parma hams**

Some types of fish

Fish is great for you and your developing baby. However, some fish may contain small amounts of pollutants, so you should limit it to two portions a week. These include oily fish like tuna, mackerel and salmon as well as other fish and seafood like turbot, sea bass and crab.

Avoid shark, swordfish and marlin because they can contain dangerous levels of mercury, and stay away from raw shellfish because that can lead to food-poisoning which could affect your health and that of your baby.

- **Do not eat shark and marlin**
- **Limit oily fish and tuna to twice a week**
- **Avoid raw shellfish such as oysters**

Coffee

Lots of women go off coffee in pregnancy. Maybe it's their body telling them something because too much caffeine has been linked to miscarriage and low birth weight babies. If you still love your latte, cut your caffeine to 200mg a day. That works out as two mugs of instant coffee, one mug of filtered coffee, two large cups of tea, or five cans of coke a day.

Alcohol

A cheeky glass of fizz to celebrate the pregnancy won't do any harm will it? Well, the truth is, the guidelines about drinking alcohol in pregnancy have evolved and changed as we've learned more about the potential impact on your unborn child. Now, the Chief Medical Officer says:

If you are pregnant or planning a pregnancy, the safest approach is not to drink alcohol at all, to keep risks to your baby to a minimum. Drinking in pregnancy can lead to long-term harm to the baby, with the more you drink the greater the risk.

There simply is no amount of alcohol that's been proven to be safe, and these guidelines make things much clearer. Some women do choose to drink. If that's you, to minimise the risks to your baby you should:

Avoid alcohol for the first three months of pregnancy. Drinking small amounts of alcohol after this time does not seem to be harmful.

- Don't drink more than one or two units at a time.
- Only drink once or twice per week.
- Never binge drink (six units or more at one time).

The trouble is, it's incredibly tricky to keep tabs on how much you're drinking. The only way to be sure your baby isn't affected by booze is to stay away.

With a little care, you can stay healthy and nourish and nurture your baby—and remember it's only nine months; you can plan a post-pregnancy picnic to enjoy the foods you've missed!

Toxoplasmosis fears

In my first pregnancy, I was concerned I could get toxoplasmosis. I'd never had it so I had no antibodies. This concern led me to fear of eating meat, touching it, or even buying it in the supermarket. I also asked my partner to be careful when handling meat. Throughout the pregnancy, I became more and more scared I could accidentally harm the baby. I also got scared of cheese, beauty products, body fluids, and much more. This fear was not just related to products I consumed but for my entire family. This led to feeling stressed and scared. The longer the pregnancy went on, the more products I got scared of. I didn't trust myself anymore. This behaviour peaked in panic attacks when I touched something by mistake that I thought could harm the baby, even when it was totally unrealistic.

~ Cheryl, London

Dr Keith says:

Toxoplasmosis is an infection by an organism called toxoplasma gondii, and it is found mainly in continental European soils. It isn't endemic in the UK, and therefore we don't screen for it. However, it is associated with birth defects, and for this reason, we don't recommend eating ham from endemic areas in case the pig has been infected and then passes it on through their meat. The organism can also be present in cat faeces, lambing ewes, newly born lambs, and root vegetables, so you should avoid close contact with animals, and I always recommend washing vegetables.

However, if your fears about your pregnancy and the wellbeing of your baby are affecting your mental health, ask your doctor for help and support.

10

WHAT HAPPENS IF YOU'RE EXPECTING TWINS?

The news that you're expecting twins can be incredibly exciting but a little scary too. The risks of the pregnancy together with the challenge of caring and providing for more than one baby can be intimidating. However, with the right support, guidance and information you can help yourself stay healthy, protect your growing babies and prepare for birth and beyond.

There's a saying that it's 'double the trouble and twice the joy.' And it's true that multiple pregnancy is associated with increased risk for both mother and babies. Maternal mortality is 2.5 times that for singleton births, and the risk of having to deliver early is also significantly higher in multiple pregnancies. Around half of all twin pregnancies are delivered before term, which can mean they need significant neonatal health support.

The good news is that assisted reproduction treatments and increasing maternal age mean that the number of multiple births has risen significantly over the last thirty years, now accounting for as many as three per cent of live births. Your obstetrician and midwife will be experienced in helping you have a healthy pregnancy and a safe delivery so your babies are protected and prepared for life.

I'm having what?

Early on, a bigger than average bump may be a clue that there could be more than one baby developing inside your womb. You may also notice more nausea and niggles in early pregnancy. You may gain a lot of weight, feel particularly tired and drained, or suffer badly with morning sickness. But the truth is that pregnancy is unpredictable; each woman responds differently to the hormonal changes and the physical demands her body is facing. None of these signs means for certain that you're expecting twins.

Mums who are pregnant with twins often notice that the line on their pregnancy test is darker and more distinct at an early stage. That's because levels of the hormone hCG (human chorionic gonadotropin) is usually elevated in multiple pregnancies. This can also be detected on blood tests. But the one sure way to positively confirm you're pregnant with twins is with your first dating ultrasound scan, when two tiny heartbeats may be visible.

Dr Keith confesses:

When I was a registrar, a woman who hadn't been booked in was brought to the hospital by ambulance, having already delivered her first baby. We gave her a drug to cause the uterus to contract, and deliver the placenta, but as we did so we realised there was another baby in there! I had to quickly give the mother some gas and air, and reach in to deliver the little one. The baby arrived into the world safely, but it was quite a surprise for Mum!

Twin types

You should be carefully scanned between eleven and fourteen weeks so the chorionicity, amnionicity and the placentas of your babies can be assessed. If those words sound unintelligible, don't worry. It's simply a way of examining the number of outer membranes (chorionic) and inner membranes (amniotic) around your babies.

Why does twin type matter?

The importance of twin typing goes well beyond whether your two babies are going to look alike. The information can help you and your medical team understand about the relative level of risk to your unborn children. Pregnancies with only one chorionic layer tend to have increased risk of transfusions between twins, growth restriction and congenital abnormalities and will need extra care and monitoring throughout pregnancy.

Dr Keith's guide to twin types

Twins can be the result of a variety of causes. They can arise due to the release of multiple eggs or multiple ovulations, the splitting of a single fertilised egg, or they can result from fertility treatments such as in vitro fertilisation (IVF), which involves the insertion of many fertilised eggs into the womb.

The particular way in which twins are conceived determines the degree of relatedness between the two little ones as well as whether they're identical or not.

Dizygotic or fraternal twins

This is the most common type of multi-fetal or twin pregnancy. It happens when two separate eggs are fertilised by two separate sperm cells. This means that dizygotic twins are like any other pair of siblings. They don't have exactly the same genetic make-up and so they do not look identical and can be different sexes.

If you're wondering how two eggs can be available for fertilisation at the same time, you're not alone. Many shell-shocked parents have asked me precisely the same question. The truth is, there are lots of different reasons.

Researchers suggest that some mothers may be genetically prone to releasing lots of eggs instead of just the one and this type of twin does tend to run in families. As well as this tendency, this can also be more likely with older mums or with the use of some fertility drugs such as clomid.

In rare, but often newsworthy cases, two eggs can be fertilised at different times by sperm from two different dads. This can result in fraternal twins with two different fathers—a tricky one to deal with both emotionally and practically.

Monozygotic or identical twins

This occurs when one fertilised egg splits in two. This means that the genetic material from the egg and the sperm are the same, producing two identical embryos.

So monozygotic twins are genetically the same sex and generally look exactly the same, or thereabouts. I say thereabouts, because although their DNA is essentially identical, environmental factors can have a significant influence on genes. They can be turned on and off in a phenomenon known as *epigenetic modification*. Even in identical twins there will be ways of telling the difference, and as someone who has delivered many, many twins I am intrigued by how two individuals with the same DNA can be so different, both physically and emotionally.

Monozygotic twinning can occur spontaneously after natural conception or after IVF treatment. Are you confused? Let's review the development of the fertilised egg. It starts when two cells, an ovum and a sperm cell combine to form a single cell called the zygote.

For reasons that are really not fully understood, the zygote may divide into two, producing identical twins. The later in pregnancy that this division occurs, the more structures that will be shared. These two blastocysts can both implant in the endometrial lining of the uterus to form two identical embryos. Even after years of studying, researching and delivering twins, it's still a process that fills me with awe.

Chorionicity

The **chorionicity** of twins relates to whether they share the same placenta and lining of the fluid sac, and is dependent on precisely when the zygote divides:

- **Dichorionic/diamniotic:** These twins divide at the earliest stage and so each twin has their own placenta as well as their own chorion and amniotic sac
- **Monochorionic/diamniotic**: The zygote forming these twins, will usually divide between four and eight days after fertilisation. These identical twins share a placenta and chorionic sac but have their own amniotic sac
- **Monochorionic/monoamniotic:** These twins develop from a zygote that splits late, usually between eight and twelve days after conception. The twins will share a placenta, chorionic and amniotic sac. If the division occurs more than twelve days after fertilisation, the twins will share even more and are likely to be conjoined and share body parts.

A healthy twin pregnancy

Eating for three, or more

If you're pregnant with more than one baby, it's especially important to look after your own health and wellbeing. A balanced diet with plenty of fruit, veg, fish, lean meat and eggs, pulses, dairy and wholegrains will nourish your body and the babies growing inside you. Exercise will keep you fit and ready for the challenges ahead, and together with quitting smoking and alcohol will ensure you give your babies the best start to life.

Boost your blood

You're more at risk from anaemia during a multiple pregnancy. Boost your body's iron levels with red meat, fortified cereals and loads of leafy green veggies washed down with a glass of orange juice. The vitamin C will help your body absorb the iron.

Down time

A multiple pregnancy can be wonderful, but it can also be utterly exhausting. Be gentle with yourself. Take regular rest, make sure you get enough sleep and if you're stressed out get some support from friends, family or your healthcare team.

Nausea and other niggles

The increased size of your bump, the demands of your growing babies and your hormonal surge can mean that a multiple pregnancy brings increased problems along with pregnancy's usual niggles and gripes.

Morning sickness and indigestion can be a real problem, so try eating little and often to stave off symptoms, and see your midwife for antacids that can safely soothe the burn.

The weight of your babies can press on your pelvic blood vessels, increasing the risk of varicose veins and piles. Stay comfortable with support tights and put your legs up when you have a quiet moment. Plenty of fluids and fibre will keep you regular and prevent painful constipation.

Your expanding bump, together with pregnancy hormones that soften and stretch your ligaments mean you may be plagued by backache or pelvic pain later in pregnancy. Don't suffer in silence. Speak to your midwife who may refer you to a specialist physiotherapist who can recommend exercises, techniques and body supports.

Antenatal care

Antenatal appointments are important in pregnancy, and that is especially true if you're carrying twins. Your doctor and midwife will want to keep a close eye on you and your babies. You will be carefully assessed and cared for by a multidisciplinary team. If you are thought to have a higher-risk or complicated multiple pregnancy, a consultant from a specialist fetal medicine centre will also give advice on your care.

If you have a multiple pregnancy, you are at increased risk of high blood pressure, gestational diabetes and preterm delivery. However, with close monitoring and treatment of any problems your team should be able to keep you and your babies as healthy as possible.

By 24 weeks your team will talk through the risks, signs and symptoms of preterm labour with you, and at 32 weeks they will expand this discussion to agree on the timing of birth and the possible mode of delivery. Together you can develop the best birth plan for you and your babies.

I was the expectant mother of girl and boy twins. I woke at one a.m. aware of a little wetness. Unable to spring up, I manoeuvred my heavy cumbersome body out of bed, and as I did so I felt a gush of water burst suddenly from me. I was surprised how clear and pure the water appeared as it formed pools on our laminate flooring. Just as quickly, I felt something flop out from within me and I had a horrid feeling that something wasn't right. What had flopped out was my unborn daughter's leg. Surprisingly, I remained calm as I told my husband to call his mum who lived around the corner to come and take care of our son who was still sleeping soundly. I had a great urge to have a poo. However, as I approached the toilet with a leg hanging out of me, I decided against this: I thought one push and I'll be giving birth in the toilet.

We drove to the hospital with me avoiding sitting down and putting any pressure on the protruding limb. I also worried that she was going to push her way out before we got to hospital and I was aware of the complications that might occur if she came out legs first.

I phoned on the way and I was pleased to see a nurse waiting for me with a wheelchair.

I had to have an emergency C-section. Soon after, I was numb from my waist down due to my epidural and I felt something close to relaxed. My twin children Harry and Hannah were born within an hour of arriving at the hospital and with only four minutes between them. I remember the moments after the births well, and the feeling of calm that pervaded. For me, this was a much less stressful experience than the natural birth of Richard, my first born.

~ Hayley, Blackpool

11

ARE THERE INCREASED RISKS FOR OLDER MOTHERS?

We use the term 'elderly primigravida' for any woman who is over thirty-five and pregnant for the first time. It's a slightly old-fashioned expression that makes lots of my patients cringe and reach for the skin serum. I don't blame them; I'm an older parent myself. With women focusing on careers and settling into relationships later, the average age of childbirth is rising markedly in Britain and across Western societies, so in many ways, it could be considered the new normal.

However, embarking on pregnancy a little later in life does bring some risks. Headlines about the dangers of miscarriage, chromosomal defects, congenital abnormalities and pregnancy hypertension can be frightening. But try not to get stressed; the risks are often exaggerated in the media. Your team will be experienced at caring for expectant mothers of all ages. With good screening, antenatal care and support you can expect to have a happy and healthy pregnancy.

First things first

Your main difficulty may be getting pregnant in the first place. Fertility starts to decrease slightly after thirty and then more dramatically after thirty-five, so you may need patience. However, reaching the age of thirty-five doesn't mean it's too late to conceive naturally. Indeed, I've cared for many older mums. But it's a good idea to get on with it, if possible.

I know this from my own experience. I met my wife, Sharon, relatively late on in my career. Although we were keen to start a family, it took a long time for her to get pregnant.

One study found that for couples having regular sex without contraception 92% of those aged 19-26 conceived after one year and 98% after two years. This dropped to 82% of 35-39 year-olds after one year and 90% after two years. So the statistics are still pretty good, and the sooner you start, the better your chances.

If you're fit and well with regular periods and in your twenties or early thirties, it's worth trying for at least year before going to see your GP. However, if you've reached thirty-five, it's better to get help a little earlier. Consider a check after six months or so if you've not fallen pregnant. However, if you have had gynaecological problems like endometriosis, your periods are irregular or you are worried about your reproductive health, it's a good idea to see your doctor for advice and assessment straight away

Screening

Your joy at seeing the blue line on your pregnancy test may be tinged with fear of abnormalities in your developing baby. Genetic and chromosomal defects occur more frequently with increasing age and the risk of having a baby with a chromosomal abnormality, such as Down's syndrome, is highest when you are over forty.

There are excellent investigations available to help identify any problems. The decision whether to have screening or diagnostic tests is personal, although your doctor or midwife will be able to advise and guide you through the maze of antenatal tests, screening and diagnostic procedures. They can also let you know about any dangers and risks associated with the tests so you can make the best choices for yourself, your family and your developing baby.

Antenatal care

I had my first pregnancy at thirty-six. I am normally an anxious person who reads too much on the internet, but my pregnancy felt right and I was content all the way through. It was so easy—I had no morning sickness, was full of energy and continued to commute to London for work until I was 38 weeks. In hospital, I was referred to as a 'geriatric mother,' which I thought was funny at thirty-six!

~ Melisssa, Brighton

Unfortunately, as a slightly older mum, you are more likely to suffer miscarriage and ectopic pregnancy. Later you may experience pregnancy complications such as high blood pressure, gestational diabetes and low-lying placenta and premature birth.

Your midwife, GP and obstetrician will be aware of potential difficulties and experienced in preventing any problems. However, although the risks are slightly increased, you are still much more likely to give birth to a healthy baby, even when you reach your mid-forties, so there is genuine cause to feel excited and optimistic.

A healthy pregnancy

By looking after yourself and altering your lifestyle you can help keep your body healthy and nurture your unborn child. Eat a nutritious balanced diet, exercise regularly and cut out cigarettes and alcohol for optimum wellbeing. The good news is that most women in their thirties tend to have healthier lifestyles than their younger counterparts, so you may already have a head start.

As always, it's essential to have regular checks. If you feel unwell with a persistent headache, exhaustion or dry mouth, or you need to nip to the loo all the time, it's important to see your doctor or midwife for a check-up.

A healthy birth

Your healthcare team will monitor you during your last weeks of pregnancy and during labour. Birth complications can occur more frequently with older mums, maybe due to the womb muscles working less efficiently, so there is an increased chance of Caesarean section and assisted deliveries.

Research also shows that although the levels are still low, there is an increased risk of stillbirth with mothers who are a little older. The reason for this isn't fully understood, but it may be linked to insufficient blood flow through the placenta and growth restriction in the unborn child. Your doctor may consider inducing labour between thirty-nine and forty weeks to prevent any problems, especially if you are over forty.

We deliver many, many healthy babies to women over thirty-five every day. The chance of these complications is small. Older mothers are often educated, settled financially and have life-experience that can prepare them well for motherhood. With the support of your team and by looking after your own health you can maintain your own wellbeing and give your baby the best start to life.

12

HOW CAN I UNDERSTAND MY MATERNITY NOTES?

Usually, your medical notes stay in a hospital storeroom or your GP's surgery, but in pregnancy it's different. You'll be given a special record book, so if you are ever in need of care, the essential information about your health and your pregnancy is carefully and clearly documented.

From your first booking appointment to your 40-week check, your midwife, your doctor, and any other health professionals who see and care for you will write down key facts and findings in your notes. You're in charge of them, so take care not to lose them because there is no back-up copy.

They're useful because as well as having your blood test results, scan findings and BP and urine readings, they also contain useful information for you, including a list of essential emergency contact numbers in case you need medical help or advice. They'll also include the details of your upcoming appointments in case baby brain has made you a little more forgetful than usual!

Err... What did you say?

I hope that when I talk to my patients, everything I say is in plain language, clear and easy to understand. However, a quick glance at your recent check-up notes will reveal a stream of abbreviations and symbols that can be incomprehensible. It's simply a type of medical shorthand, and the result of a career spent scribbling too quickly. Don't panic. I speak fluent healthcare and can help you translate the language so you can fully understand your notes. Once you get the hang of the lingo, you'll be fluent too.

> *Some things on the maternity notes were a bit confusing at times, such as results of tests etc. The good thing was that I knew if I asked my midwife, she would explain the areas I didn't understand.*
>
> **~ Sam, Northfields**

Your quick glance glossary

- **BP**: blood pressure
- **Br**: your baby is in the breech or bottom down position
- **Ceph or C or Vx**: your baby is in the head down position
- **Cx**: short for cervix, the neck of the womb
- **DNA**: did not attend; maybe baby brain is making you forgetful
- **EDD**: expected date of delivery
- **FBC**: full blood count, often done to check for anaemia
- **Fe**: this is the chemical symbol for iron and may be used if you've been given supplements to treat anaemia
- **FMF**: fetal movements have been felt
- **FMNF**: fetal movements have not been felt
- **FHH**: fetal heartbeat was heard
- **FHNH**: fetal heartbeat was not heard

- **Fundal height**: the measurement from the pubic bone to the top of the womb, usually given in centimetres
- **GTT**: glucose tolerance test given to check whether you may be developing gestational diabetes
- **Hb**: haemoglobin; this could indicate blood in the urine or the results of a blood test
- **IGT**: impaired glucose tolerance; this could indicate you may be developing gestational diabetes
- **LMP**: the first day of your last menstrual period, useful for calculating your due date
- **MSU**: mid-stream sample of your urine
- **Multigravida or multi ip**: this means you have been pregnant before, including previous miscarriages and pregnancy losses
- **NAD**: nothing abnormal is detected
- **Oed**: the presence of swelling or oedema
- **Para (with a number)**: the number of pregnancies you have had that have gone beyond 24 weeks
- **PET**: pre-eclampsia, a potentially serious condition in which the blood pressure becomes dangerously high
- **Primigravida or primip**: someone who is pregnant for the first time
- **TCA**: to come again, time to make another appointment
- **TR or trace**: tiny amounts of substances such as glucose, protein or blood have been found in your urine.
- **VE**: vaginal examination for detecting what stage you are in labour

Your baby's position

Your baby's position and presentation will be recorded. Different professionals may use varying versions of the shorthand, so we've listed them all, just in case:

Presentation: head down, bottom down or all-over the place?

- **Ceph** or **C** or **Vx**: your baby is in the head down position
- **Br**: your baby is breech or bottom down
- **Long**: your baby is lying longitudinally or vertically
- **Tr** or **Trans**: your baby is transverse or lying across your body
- **Obl**: your baby's lie is oblique or diagonally across your body

Later in pregnancy, your doctor or midwife may also identify which direction your baby's head is facing. L or R written in front of abbreviations refers to the side of your body your baby is lying on:

- **OA**: *occiput anterior*, meaning the baby is facing your back
- **OP**: *occiput posterior*, the baby is facing your front (this is also referred to as back to back or face to pubes)
- **OL**: *occiput lateral* in which the baby's head is down and facing your side

Engagement

Engagement is definitely not about your marital status. Instead, it'll tell you what proportion of your baby's head is lying in your pelvis.

- **NE/NEng/Not Eng**: your baby's head is not engaged in your pelvis
- **E/Eng**: your baby's head is engaged
- **Free**: your baby's head is still lying above your pelvis and is bobbing around freely

- **1/5-4/5**: describes how much of the head is in your pelvis. Your baby's considered to be engaged when 3/5 of their head is in your pelvis

Your baby's movements and heartbeat

You'll be keeping a close eye on your baby's movements and your midwife will monitor them too. They will also listen to the heartbeat using a trumpet or a Doppler device.

- **FMF**: fetal movements have been felt
- **FMNF**: fetal movements have not been felt
- **FHH**: the fetal heartbeat was heard
- **FHNH**: the fetal heartbeat was not heard

Your urine test

At every antenatal appointment, your midwife or doctor will perform a dip test on your urine to check for the presence of protein, glucose and blood. They're testing for glucose, which may suggest pregnancy diabetes, protein, which may indicate preeclampsia or infection and blood, which can also signal infection.

- **Alb**: stands for albumin, a protein that could indicate a potential problem such as pre-eclampsia or a urine infection
- **Pr**: this may also be used to indicate protein in the urine
- **Gluc/G**: sugar in the urine
- **Hb**: blood in the urine
- **Tr**: this refers to a small trace of protein or glucose being found
- **+/++/+++**: plus signs are used to indicate the amount of the substance in the urine. The more +, the more there is.

Your blood pressure

Your blood pressure or **BP** will be measured at every appointment. Everyone has a level that is normal for them but to give you some indication the average reading for women is around 110/70.

We consider readings above 130/90 to be high, but if you usually run a low BP we may keep a close eye on you at a level below that.

- **Oed**: indicates the presence of swelling or oedema
- **+, ++, +++**: the more plus signs, the greater the swelling

Hopefully, that's helped make everything clear. If not, don't be afraid to ask. They're your notes and it's your pregnancy. Your healthcare team will be happy to answer any questions or queries.

To be honest, I didn't really look at my maternity notes much. I did make out a birth plan in the appropriate section, but I don't know if it was even looked at! Everything is recorded, and I think because you see so many different doctors through antenatal appointments, it is for their benefit to track progress.

~ Lindsey, Kilkeel

I had a really bad experience in pregnancy as my midwife told me nothing. She handed me a folder and said to bring it with me every appointment. That was it. When I took the folder to hospital, they opened it and asked for my birthing plan. I didn't know I had to write one or what that meant. My midwife hadn't told me about any classes, so I hadn't been to any. It was so frustrating.

~ Nadine, Liverpool

13

WHAT HAPPENS IN AN ANTENATAL CHECK-UP?

When you find out you're pregnant it's natural to feel excitement and also a little apprehension about the journey ahead. Don't worry, you are not alone. From your first visit through birth and beyond, you will have regular check-ups to make sure you and your baby remain healthy and well. They're also your opportunity to ply your expert healthcare team for information and address any questions and concerns you may have.

You will be given an antenatal appointment schedule for regular check-ups, but don't forget you can get in touch with your doctor or midwife between regular checks if you have any problems or worries.

Antenatal appointment schedule

If there are no problems or complications, your antenatal appointments should follow a regular pattern. However, it's important to be aware that there may be extra check-ups if you or your baby need a little extra care. You can also ask for further appointments if you have any concerns.

When	What appointment	What happens?
As soon as you spot that thin blue line	First contact with doctor or midwife	This is your first contact with your healthcare team, when your booking appointment will be arranged.
8 to 12 weeks	Booking appointment	At your booking appointment, your doctor or midwife will find out about your medical and pregnancy history. It's your opportunity to find out about antenatal care, birth options and the screening tests you can have. You will have blood tests done, your urine and blood pressure will be checked and your dating scan will be booked.
8 to 14 weeks:	Dating scan	Your dating scan will give you a better idea of when your baby is due. It will also check its physical development and screen for possible abnormalities including Down's syndrome.
16 weeks	Routine antenatal check	Your midwife or doctor will check your blood pressure, urine and carry out blood tests to test for anaemia. They should talk through the results of any screening tests and give you information about the ultrasound scan to look for any abnormalities. This will usually be offered over the next few weeks.
18-20 weeks:	Anomaly scan	The sonographer will check that the organs have developed properly, exclude any abnormalities, locate the placental position, and they may also be able to tell you the sex of your baby.
25 weeks	Routine antenatal check	You will only have an appointment if this is your first baby. Your midwife or doctor will use a tape measure to measure the size of your uterus, measure your blood pressure and test your urine for protein.

When	What appointment	What happens?
28 weeks	Routine antenatal check	Your midwife or doctor will measure the size of your womb, check your blood pressure and test your urine for protein and glucose. You should be checked again for anaemia and an iron supplement may be given if your levels are low. If you're rhesus negative, you may be given an injection of anti-D at this time.
31 weeks	Routine antenatal check	You will have an appointment if this is your first baby. Your midwife or doctor will chat through the results of any tests from your last appointment as well as use a tape measure to measure the size of your uterus, check your blood pressure and test your urine for protein and glucose.
34 weeks	Routine antenatal check	Your midwife or doctor will give you lots of information about preparing for childbirth, including pain relief, your birth plan and how to know when you're in labour. They should also check the size of your womb, measure your blood pressure, dip your urine and review the results of any tests. If you're rhesus negative you may be offered another injection of anti-D at this time.
36 weeks	Routine antenatal check	Your midwife or doctor should give you information about breastfeeding, caring for your baby, the vitamin K that will be given at birth and any screening tests for your little one. They'll also check the size of your womb, measure your blood pressure, dip your urine and review the results of any tests.

When	What appointment	What happens?
38 weeks	Routine antenatal check	Your midwife or doctor will talk through what will happen if your pregnancy goes over 41 weeks. They'll also do the usual antenatal checks; measure the size of your womb, test your blood pressure and dip your urine for protein and glucose.
40 weeks	Routine check	You will have an appointment at 40 weeks if this is your first baby. They'll give you plenty of information about what will happen if labour doesn't start naturally in the next week. They'll measure the size of your womb, check your blood pressure and test your urine for protein and glucose as well as listening to your baby's heartbeat.
41 weeks	Post-term check	Your midwife or doctor will see you this week. They'll perform the usual checks and they'll also discuss your options and choices for induction of labour. They may also offer you a membrane sweep to kick off labour.

What happens at antenatal appointments?

Your appointments will usually take place in your local surgery, clinic or obstetrician's consulting rooms. The first booking appointment can be detailed, with lots of questions about your health, medical and family history and your lifestyle. You'll also be given an enormous amount of information about a healthy pregnancy and birth options, and there'll be plenty of chance to ask questions. This first appointment can take up to an hour, so make sure you feed the parking meter! Later appointments tend to be shorter and snappier, usually only ten to fifteen minutes, unless you have any particular symptoms or problems.

Booking appointment

Whether it's with a consultant obstetrician like myself, or with your doctor or midwife, the first booking appointment really can make pregnancy seem official. You'll get your antenatal notes and have the chance to find out more about your pregnancy care. It can be overwhelming and you may find that the questions you wanted to ask fly out of your head. I recommend that my patients make a list to help them remember.

What will happen?

Your doctor or midwife will ask lots of questions about your lifestyle, your medical history, any previous pregnancies, any medication you're taking and how you've been feeling. They will also want to know about any illnesses or genetic conditions that run in your family. Don't worry, it's more of a chat than an interrogation, but some women do find the questioning a little intrusive. It is important though, because it lets your antenatal care team understand any risks you and your baby might have. This can help identify problems rapidly so you can have the best care.

Checks and measures

Your height and weight may be measured at your booking appointment. This is to calculate your body mass index (BMI). It will usually not be checked again throughout your pregnancy, unless you're over or underweight. The ideal BMI for pregnancy is somewhere between 20 and 25. Your midwife or doctor will also check your blood pressure and test your urine.

Antenatal screening blood test

You will be offered blood tests to see if you have any conditions that might affect your health, your pregnancy and the development of your baby. These may include:

- Screening for HIV, syphilis and hepatitis B
- Blood group
- Rhesus disease
- Anaemia
- Gestational diabetes, if you are at risk
- Sickle cell and thalassaemia screening, if you're at risk

Information and advice

You'll be given plenty of information on diet, foods to avoid in pregnancy, supplements, staying fit, kicking any bad habits, and dealing with the stress, sickness and side-effects that early pregnancy can bring.

It can be a lot to take in, but hopefully this book and the articles on Your Pregnancy Doctor can help if you forget anything. But the booking appointment isn't just for your healthcare team to find out about you. It's also your opportunity to find out about antenatal care, birth options, breastfeeding and the screening tests you can have.

Scans and screening

Your midwife or doctor should let you know about the available screening tests and scans and make sure you understand what is involved.

Diet and supplements:

Ideally, you started taking a 400mcg folic acid supplement as soon as you stopped your contraception. It's proven to help protect your baby against spina bifida and other neural tube defects. The sooner you start, the better, so your midwife or doctor will check you're getting what you need. Lots of us are also deficient in vitamin D, so a supplement is recommended for all pregnant women.

Explore your emotions

Your doctor or midwife will monitor your mental as well as your physical health and should also ask about your mood. This is because pregnancy is a time of stress as well as joy. Depression is more common during the nine months as well as after the birth. If you're feeling fine, try not to feel upset about these questions. By being aware of any low mood, you can get the extra support you need so you don't sink into depression.

Free prescriptions and dental care

Every pregnant woman in the UK is entitled to free NHS dental care during pregnancy and for one year after the baby is born. Dental treatment can be expensive and your teeth and gums are vulnerable during pregnancy, so take advantage of this opportunity and book a check-up as soon as you can.

Prescriptions for medication are also free when you're pregnant and for one year after the birth in England (those living in Scotland, Wales and Northern Ireland already have free prescriptions). You simply have to fill out an FW8 Maternity Exemption form which your doctor or midwife should give you at your booking appointment.

Follow-up appointments

The rest of the antenatal appointments usually follow a similar pattern. This will include:

- A chat to check you are well and discuss any health niggles or difficulties you have.
- A blood pressure measurement to check for pre-eclampsia.
- A urine test to look for blood, protein and glucose. These can be an indication of infection, pre-eclampsia and gestational diabetes.
- Your bump will be examined and the height of the fundus measured with a tape measure to assess your baby's growth, the amount of fluid and later in pregnancy they will assess the baby's position.
- They may listen to the baby's heartbeat with a stethoscope or Doppler device.
- The results of any blood tests and screening tests will be given.
- Further tests, screening and scans will be booked and you will be talked through any risks and the potential implication of the results.

My antenatal appointments were good. Short but good. My GP organised scans and tests in the early stages, and with my second pregnancy, I was consultant-led due to having had a previous section. The doctors talked through options clearly and didn't put pressure on either way. They took plenty of time to take measurements of baby—but perhaps one downfall was that some doctors weren't great at chatting you through what they were looking for.

~ Lindsey, Kilkeel

The antenatal checks helped me feel reassured that my baby was OK. When there were issues, I was referred to the hospital to get checked over. I felt they cared for me as a patient, and always answered any questions I had. The fact you have an assigned midwife who knows about your care, as opposed to seeing different people, helps you build a nice relationship with your midwife so you feel comfortable with her.

~ Sam, Northfields

Regular appointments can help maintain your wellbeing and monitor the health of your baby. If any complications do arise, they can be quickly picked up and controlled to reduce any potential risks.

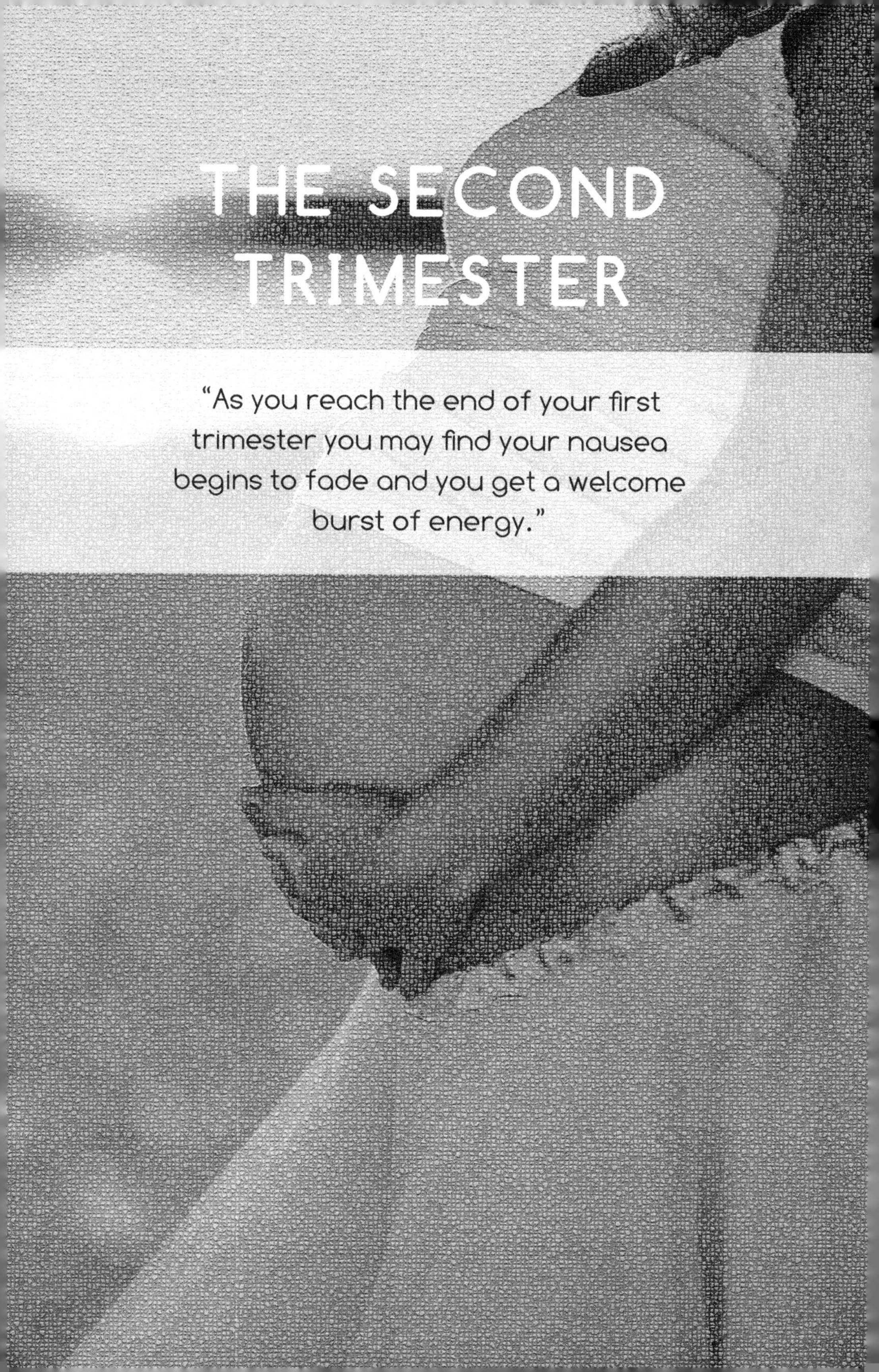

THE SECOND TRIMESTER

"As you reach the end of your first trimester you may find your nausea begins to fade and you get a welcome burst of energy."

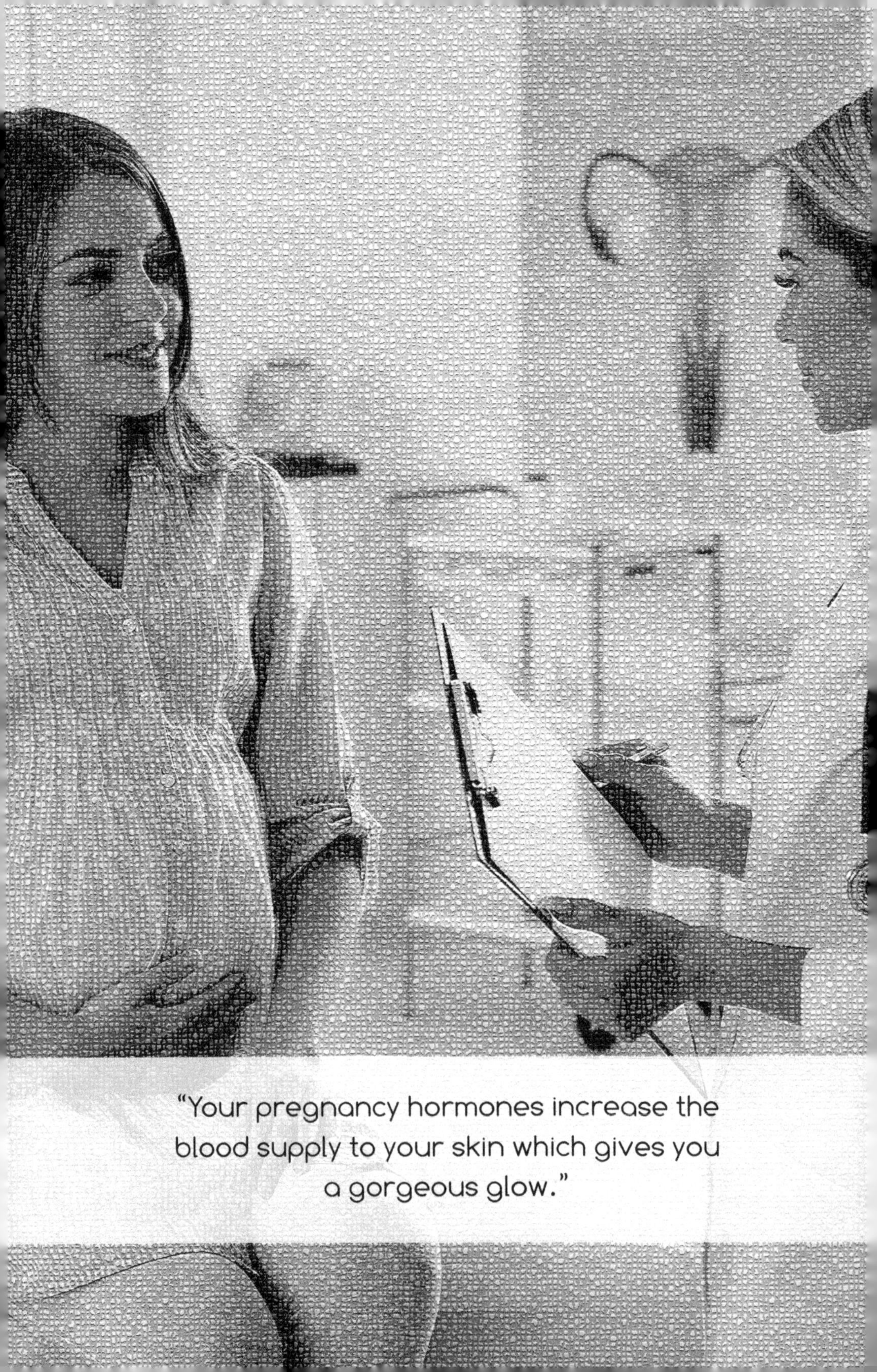

"Your pregnancy hormones increase the blood supply to your skin which gives you a gorgeous glow."

14

WHEN WILL I START TO BLOOM?

During the second trimester lots of women start to breathe a sigh of relief and decide to go public with their pregnancy. This is because a miscarriage becomes much less likely after this stage, so it's a wonderful milestone to reach.

That's not the only good news; as you reach the end of the first trimester you may find your fatigue gradually fades and you get a welcome burst of energy. Plus, most women find their queasiness dies down in the fourth month and they can really start to bloom and enjoy their pregnancy.

But if you're not feeling beautiful and blooming, please don't stress. There's such a pressure on women to feel fabulous in pregnancy but lots of women don't. Nausea can be ongoing and many women suffer with prenatal depression. If you're struggling, see your doctor or midwife for support and treatment.

Your skin in pregnancy

Pregnant women on Instagram and in magazines often look golden and glowing. It's true that some lucky women sail through pregnancy with perfect skin, but for many there are pimples and pigmentation, stretchmarks and itching.

Blushing and blooming

In pregnancy, the blood volume increases, so there's more pumping around your body. Hormones also increase the blood supply to your skin, which may give you a gorgeous peachy glow. If that's you, count your lucky stars. It can make lots of women hot, bothered, flushed and ruddy faced.

Spot stress

Your pregnancy hormones can really change your skin. The rampaging hormones can also trigger the pimples and pustules you thought you'd left behind at puberty. Acne can be miserable, really knocking your confidence and self-esteem. Try our self-help tips but please, don't be afraid to see your doctor for guidance and treatment. There are great medications for spots and lots are still safe to use in pregnancy. You don't have to put up with bad skin.

What can I do?

- Cleanse your skin regularly with a gentle product that won't strip your skin of oils.
- Use a light oil-free moisturiser that won't clog and congest.
- Don't scrub: Be kind to your skin to prevent irritation, use your hands to wash gently and pat dry.
- Don't pick and prod: Squeezing, popping and poking will make things worse. It's a sure-fire way of increasing inflammation and causing scarring. Step away from the magnifying mirror.

- Cover-up: If your skin is affecting your confidence, try some concealer. Modern products are so much better than the orange blobs you may have seen in the past. Pick non-comedogenic products to prevent break-outs, and cleanse carefully before bed.
- Get help: Talk to your doctor, midwife or pharmacist for lotions and potions that are safe in pregnancy.
- Don't beg, borrow or steal a friend's spot remedy. Lots of skin products (including retinoic acid and retinols) contain ingredients that are related to vitamin A. They are used in skin preparations and creams to fight acne and the effects of aging. They can be effective but they are not safe in pregnancy because they can cause developmental problems in the unborn child.

> *I had terrible acne from my teenage years and I'd controlled it with the pill, so I was terrified about breaking out in pregnancy. In fact, my skin was amazing, I don't know about blooming but it wasn't red and bumpy, which was way better than it had ever been before. I think the hormones really suited me, Sadly, three months after the birth the pimples were back with a vengeance.*
>
> **~ Jane, Leeds**

Patchy pigmentation

As many as ninety per cent of women notice darker pigmentation in pregnancy. This can affect your nipples which can turn from pink to brown. Your skin can also darken around the tummy button and in a line down to your pubic bone, the **linea nigra**.

The pigmentation increases in sunlight and tanning can often be a little patchy. Some women develop an area of skin darkening on the central part of the face. This is called the *mask of pregnancy* or **chloasma faciei**.

The pigmentation often fades with time but you can help to keep your skin evenly coloured and blooming.

Dr Keith says:

- Always wear a high protection sunscreen.
- Avoid intense sunlight.
- Cover-up: Wear cool clothing in natural fibres, slip on a hat, or even rock out a parasol. Anything to keep your skin safely shaded.

Itchy skin

Itching is common in pregnancy and is thought to be caused by a combination of the skin stretching and the hormone oestrogen. It's often worse in summer pregnancies, when prickly heat can have you tearing at the skin on your tummy.

What can I do?

- Wear loose cotton clothing to stay cool and comfortable.
- Massage oil or cream into your bump to soothe your skin and get in touch with your growing baby.
- Try adding bicarbonate of soda or oatmeal to your bath water. They're cheaper than bubble bath and really ease itching skin.

When to get help

Severe, widespread itching in the last few months of pregnancy, particularly if you are feeling unwell or have become jaundiced, could indicate the rare complication **cholestasis of pregnancy**.

Cholestasis is a liver condition which affects less than one in a thousand pregnancies. It is potentially dangerous because it may be associated with stillbirth or maternal bleeding after birth. It is important to contact your doctor if you have severe itching, yellowing of the eyes, or have noticed your urine is dark or your stools are unusually pale.

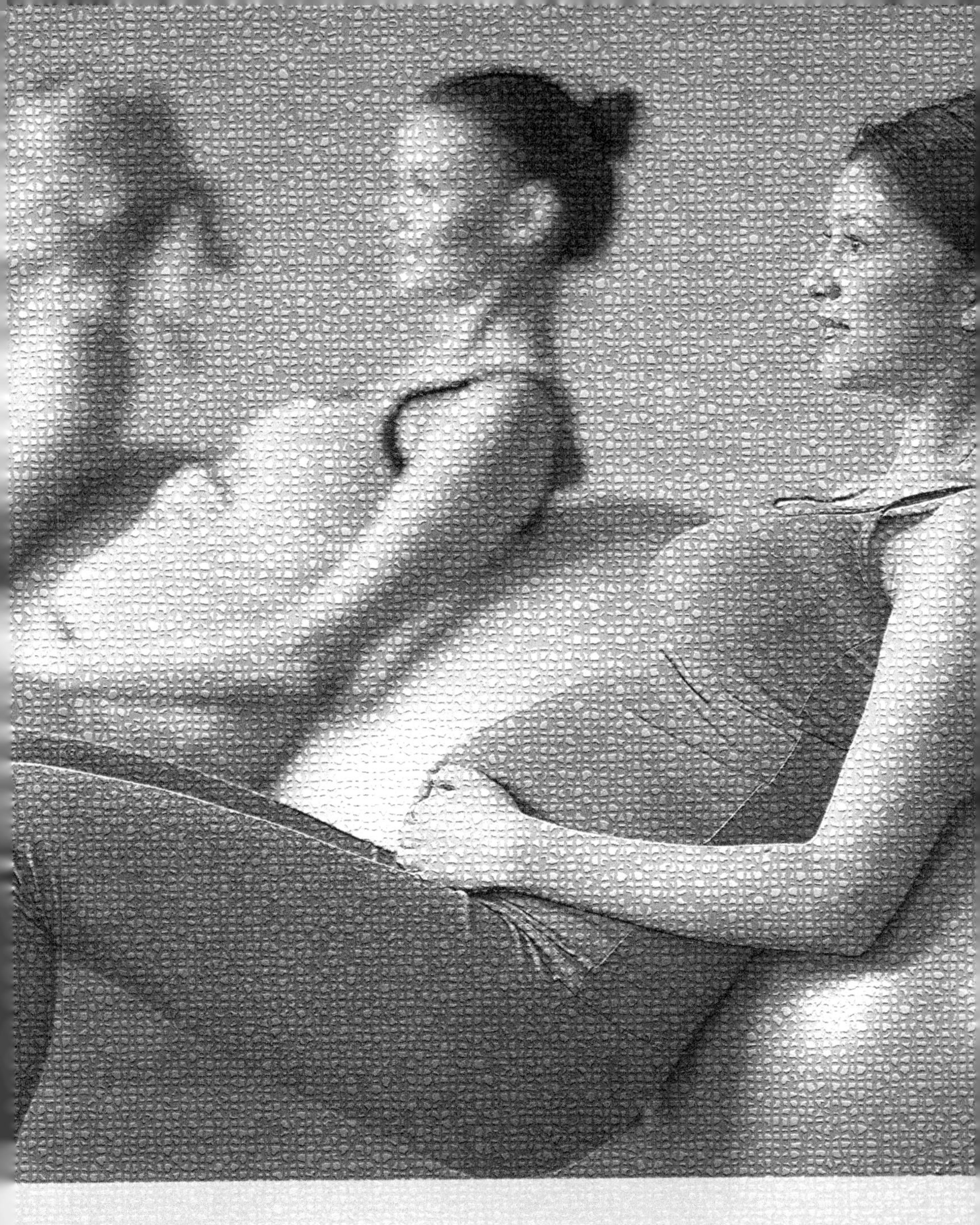

"Exercise is great during pregnancy but listen to your body. If you begin to feel any pain, dizziness or nausea it's time to rest and recover."

15

IS IT SAFE TO EXERCISE IN PREGNANCY?

Exercise can make you feel good, improve your health and protect against obesity and gestational diabetes. However, your body changes, your growing bump and the flood of hormones mean it's not always safe to exercise in the same way you used to. That doesn't mean you should slump on the sofa. With a little care you can get moving so you'll be fit and ready for the challenges of childbirth.

Check your health

It's important to chat to your doctor or midwife before starting or changing an exercise regime. If you've worked-out regularly and there are no problems with your pregnancy, chances are you'll be able to continue to exercise with a few modifications. However, sometimes exercise is not safe and could put you or your baby at risk. It's essential to stop exercising and get medical attention if you suffer:

- Vaginal bleeding
- Dizziness, faintness or headache
- Chest pain or increasing shortness of breath

- Palpitations, an uneven or fast heartbeat
- Contractions that continue after you have rested for a while
- Fluid leaking from your vagina
- Decreased fetal movements
- Calf pain or swelling (this could indicate a thrombosis in the deep veins of the legs)

Listen to your body

Your body should tell you when you're doing too much. If it's starting to protest, or if you feel any pain, weakness or dizziness, it's time to rest and recover. It's fine to feel a little puffed, but don't exercise to the point of exhaustion. You should have enough breath to keep chatting throughout. If you don't, cut down the intensity.

Dr Keith says:

Many of the women I care for are active and exercise in pregnancy. They seem to manage well until around 24 weeks, when they often need to change to a gentler, low impact regime.

Food for fuel

Your body is working hard to build your baby and that process needs plenty of fuel and nourishment. Exercise burns calories, so make sure you eat enough to compensate.

Warm up

A gentle warm-up gets your muscles, joints and your heart-rate going so they're ready for the challenges ahead. The pregnancy hormones make your ligaments soft and stretchy, which can make your joints vulnerable to injury. If you skip the warm-up, you're more likely to end up with painful aches and strains.

A good trick is to start off doing your chosen exercise at a low intensity for the first five minutes. It lets your body know what's ahead, so it adapts and prepares for more vigorous activity.

Stay hydrated

In pregnancy, your metabolism is up, your body's working harder and your kidneys are doing overtime. All of that, combined with exercise, can mean you're at risk of dehydration. Keep drinking water throughout your exercise session and afterwards. Your wee should be pale straw coloured. If it's dark yellow or gold, keep sipping water.

Dehydration isn't good for you or your baby. If it's severe, the blood flow to the placenta could decrease. It can also increase your risk of fainting, overheating, or even going into early labour.

Go slow

If you're lying down, get up slowly to allow your blood-pressure to adapt. Rushing things can lead to dizziness, fainting and falls. Be aware that your changing body shape and growing bump can alter your centre of gravity—it can take a while to get used to the new you. Often, women can be a little clumsy and off-balance. Take care when you change position so you stay stable and safe.

Cool down

The cool down is as important as the warm-up but it's the bit that's most often missed as everyone flocks to the showers or the café. At the end of your workout, continue to exercise at a low intensity for five minutes. This can be a gentle walk or whatever floats your boat. Afterwards do some gentle stretching to prevent soreness and stiff muscles.

Get in the habit

Don't make the mistake of exercising too hard, too soon. It's much better to commit to a regular, manageable exercise routine you can stick to. Exercising with friends can be a great way of dragging yourself out when you'd rather snuggle under the duvet. Recruit a mate so you can have fun and stay motivated.

I tried to keep healthy, but didn't attempt to do anything I wasn't used to. Towards the end I used to walk a lot as I was hoping it would help me go into labour, as I was late with both pregnancies.

~ Sam, Northfields

I really enjoyed exercising during pregnancy and definitely felt it kept me more mobile and energised especially in the last trimester. However, I did suffer from some pelvic pain and this was sometimes aggravated by certain exercises, especially squats and lunges, so be careful!

When I returned to exercise after having my baby I went for it a hundred per cent, which was a bit of a mistake as I had undiagnosed diastasis recti and ended up giving myself a hernia where my muscles were still separated. Ask your doctor to give you the once over at your six-week check. It will speed up the healing process and avoid any nasty injuries!

~ Sarah, Larne

Exercise that isn't safe in pregnancy

There are some activities you should avoid, no matter how fit and fearless you are:

Unsafe sports

Stay safe when you exercise and that means giving dangerous sports a miss. You may be a brilliant skier, gymnast, showjumper or mountain biker, but accidents happen to the best. A fall or crash could put you and your baby at risk. For the same reason, it's a good idea to avoid sports that involve lots of contact and shoving like rugby, or even netball, if you play at a high level.

Road cycling should be safe in early pregnancy, so long as you feel comfortable and don't push it too far. Later on, when your bump may throw you off balance, it's sensible to stick to life cycle and spin classes.

If you play a mean game of tennis, it's probably safe to continue. But if you're new to racket sports, pregnancy is not a good time to start. The quick movements, arm swings and direction changes could leave you going head over heels.

Scuba diving should be avoided in pregnancy. Your baby simply isn't protected from the dramatic changes in pressure and it may affect their development.

Flat out

After the first trimester, it's not a good idea to lie flat on your back. The womb can press down on the vena cava (the vein that sends blood back to your heart). Your blood supply can fall, leaving you weak, dizzy and short of breath. If you're doing Pilates, yoga or conditioning, let your teacher know about your pregnancy so they can adapt the exercises to suit your needs. Popping a cushion or a foam wedge under your upper back can really help. It'll prop you up a little so you are almost flat and can exercise safely and in comfort.

Easy does it

Pregnancy is a time to be kind and gentle to your body. Even if you were a fitness fiend before, it's important to take things a little easier. Your body should be your guide; listen to it and respond to any pain or problems.

Stay cool

Your baby is your own in-built central heating system. The increased blood flow and metabolic rate in pregnancy can make you hot and bothered. Exercise can pump up your temperature more, so take it easy, avoid hot and humid conditions and choose cool, breathable workout wear. Stay well away from steamy activities like Bikram or Hot Yoga and relax with a tepid shower, not the sauna or hot tub.

If you've overdone it, you may feel warm, sick, dizzy and unwell. Rest immediately and strip off some layers. Sit somewhere air-conditioned and sip cold water to cool and rehydrate.

Exercises every woman should do

Before pregnancy, you probably took your pelvic floor for granted. It was just there, doing its job, surrounding and supporting the organs in your pelvis. But those pesky pregnancy hormones can loosen the muscles of the pelvic floor. This, together with your growing womb pressing on your bladder can lead to urine leaking, especially when you cough, sneeze or laugh. Childbirth can further stretch and weaken things, so if you don't want to rely on popping a pad in your pants every day, it's a good idea to start working on your pelvic floor now.

Where is my pelvic floor?

Your pelvic floor is made up of the muscles around the womb, bowels and bladder. Think of them as a sling, keeping everything supported and in place. There's an easy trick to help you identify the muscles and learn how to control them. When you next have a wee, try to stop the flow for a couple of seconds. The muscles you're clenching are the muscles of the pelvic floor.

That's not the ideal way to exercise them, though. All that stopping mid-flow is a little uncomfortable and if repeated could lead to a urinary tract infection. Instead, follow my exercise regime to build up strength, help it bounce back after childbirth, improve your sex life and prevent leaks.

How do I exercise my pelvic floor muscles?

Now you know how to tense the muscles, you can do it when you're not on the loo. Work on tightening and lifting the whole area; it's like stopping a wee, gripping a tampon and holding in a poo, all at the same time! Try to do a mixture of quick clenches and long, slow squeezes for maximum benefit.

- **Quick clench**: Pull in your pelvic floor quickly, tightening and squeezing the muscles upwards. Pause and slowly relax, then repeat.

- **Slow squeeze**: Slowly tighten and lift the pelvic floor. Think of it as an elevator slowly moving up through your pelvis and into your tummy. Hold it for 1, 2, 3, 4 seconds then slowly release, letting that elevator slowly return to the ground floor and repeat. You may struggle to manage four seconds when you first start, so build up the hold time, keeping a little in reserve to allow you to gradually relax and not let it flop at the end of the exercise.

Practise at home and check you're not doing strange things to your face as you concentrate on the contractions. Then you can do them any time, any place, anywhere. It's a good idea to pick something to trigger your memory. Put a sticker on your mirror to remind you to exercise while you're brushing your teeth, do them whenever you pop the kettle on, when you're on the bus or sitting at traffic lights.

Try to do a mixture of quick clenches and slow squeezes five times a day. Start off with five squeezes and build up to ten when you're strong enough. Why don't you start now? Go on, flex that floor.

16

I'M HAPPY TO BE PREGNANT. WHY DO I FEEL SO DOWN?

Post-natal depression is talked about a lot. You may read about women who've been through it, or see stories on TV. In contrast, prenatal depression is not often discussed—in fact, the time before the birth is portrayed as being full of joy and anticipation. But I've seen in my practice that for many, many women this is not the case. Pregnancy can be a time filled with stress, anxiety and depression.

Research shows us that depression is becoming more and more common in young women. In many ways, it's not surprising that at a time of huge emotional and physical change, as many as one in five women can be affected by the illness.

Sadly, lots of pregnant women suffer in silence. They may be confused at their lack of elation and afraid to get help because they feel guilty or ashamed of their feelings of sadness. Depression is an illness, both in pregnancy and outside it. You are not to blame. There are effective treatments available and ways in which you can boost your mood. If these signs and symptoms are striking a chord with you, seek out help and support today.

Am I depressed?

Pregnancy is a time of change, in your life and in your body. Many women blame their depressed mood on being hormonal. It's true that some of the signs of depression can be found in pregnancy; lots of women feel exhausted and lacking in energy, many may struggle with sleep-disturbance and appetite changes. But if you're feeling overwhelmingly sad or anxious to the extent that it's affecting your life, your wellbeing and your relationships, you should get help.

Women who are depressed during pregnancy will usually suffer from some of these symptoms for many days for a period of at least two weeks:

- Feeling sad persistently and for prolonged periods. Many depressed women are more tearful than normal, but some may feel flat and almost emotionless.
- Feeling worthless, guilty or inadequate.
- Having recurring thoughts of hopelessness and worthlessness. Some women may also think about death or even suicide.
- Experiencing ongoing and sometimes overwhelming feelings of anxiety, worry and panic.
- Having difficulty leaving the house, mixing with friends and colleagues or dealing with social situations.
- Being grouchy and irritable with your partner, your children, the man at the bus-stop, the woman at the supermarket check-out—frankly, anyone can trigger these feelings.
- Having difficulty concentrating and focusing on things. This may make you forgetful and absent minded.
- Sleeping much more than normal, or struggling to get the sleep you need. Some people may wake in the early hours of the morning and find it difficult to drop back off. Worrying and obsessing about problems in the wee, small hours is also common.

- Losing motivation and interest in activities you usually find enjoyable.
- Having a change in appetite so you lose interest in food, don't enjoy your meals or sometimes eat more food as a source of comfort.

Untreated depression can affect you and your baby. When you're down, it can be difficult to look after yourself properly and get the nutrition you need. Women with depression are also more likely to blunt their feelings with alcohol, drugs and cigarettes. Babies born to depressed mums may be less active and more agitated, so it's important to get help for both of your sakes.

I've got nothing to be depressed about

Depression during pregnancy is a biological illness. It isn't you being weak or ungrateful, it's about changes in your brain chemistry. It affects between one in five and one in ten pregnant women, with many more struggling without treatment because they feel ashamed about their feelings.

The hormonal changes of pregnancy can alter the balance of chemicals in your brain and affect your mood. This can be made worse by the physical exhaustion of pregnancy and the stress that such a big life change can have on your life, your relationship and your finances.

The rise and rise of social media has also piled the pressure on pregnant women. You're bombarded with images of perfect people, blooming with health and displaying gorgeous, neat, little, bumps. The farting, belching, stretch-marked reality can be tough to take.

Believe me, you're not alone with your feelings and your fears. There are ways to boost your mood. With help and support you can come out of this dark cloud, start to enjoy your pregnancy and look forward to the birth with optimism and hope.

Helping yourself through depression

Talk it out

A problem shared really is a problem, if not halved, definitely significantly reduced. Opening up to friends, family and your partner can reduce your stress and fear. Your emotions are not a dirty secret to be ashamed of. Talking to others can defuse tension and help you view problems from another perspective.

Light it up

Sunlight really can make your spirits soar. The short dark days really can make us sad as well as SAD. Get out into the open air every day. Choose lunchtime when the sun is at its highest and feel the light lift your mood.

Make a list

Making a list of what you need to do and ticking them off can help you celebrate every little achievement. Don't overface yourself, it'll bring you down. Instead, set small achievable goals and be kind to yourself if you slip up.

Mood food

When you're down, it's easy to grab sweet, stimulating foods for a quick boost. But sugar, caffeine and fast-food highs quickly fade, leaving your blood sugar levels depressed and your mood even lower. Instead, you should choose complex slow release carbs like wholegrains and pulses, plenty of fruit and leafy green vegetables, and healthy fats from fish, avocado and nuts to nourish your body.

It makes a difference. A survey by the Food and Mood project, led by the mental health charity Mind, showed that around 90% of people found that changing their diet significantly improved their mental health.

Be positive

It's too easy to get into a negative mindset, with your brain going over and over bad or sad images and imagining terrible scenarios. Stop the bad stuff. It's not real, it's your brain playing tricks on you. Try to picture positive images, a happy baby, you peacefully breastfeeding, walking with a pram in a beautiful park. Practise positive visualisation, and if you start to dwell on scary or negative stuff, try exercising, reading or phoning a friend to break the cycle.

Practise mindfulness

You don't need me to tell you that your life is changing dramatically. Thinking too much about that can be scary and overwhelming. Instead of going over and over any worries in your mind, try to stay in the moment. Focus on what's happening right now. It'll ease your stress and anxiety and the exercises are brilliant for using during labour too.

Try concentrating your full attention on your breathing following the air in and out. Really focus on the sound and feel of the air going in and out, releasing your negative thoughts and feelings.

Get moving

You probably want to curl up into a ball, but physical activity can stimulate the release of the body's happy hormones, endorphins, which can decrease pain, give a sense of wellbeing and help you get the sleep you need. They're like your own safe, in-built opiate.

But it's not just this feel-good hormone that is boosted. Exercise may also raise the amount of serotonin in the brain. Most modern antidepressants work by upping serotonin levels, so exercise can work in the same way and decrease symptoms of depression and anxiety. It's difficult. but it will make a difference.

Support groups

Often, talking about your situation with other people can help, especially if you can share with people who are going through the same thing. Friends and family can be a great support practically and emotionally, but sometimes speaking to someone who is unconnected to your family unit can really be of benefit.

Guided self-help

This is a treatment based on cognitive behavioural therapy. It can help people suffering from anxiety, depression and stress. It is based on research evidence and uses a positive, problem-solving approach to change the way you feel and act. Several self-help sessions are held with a therapist, either in person, online or over the phone. You can continue the process as 'homework'.

Getting help for depression

Make an appointment to see your doctor. Be totally honest and open about your feelings. Your GP will understand because they will have seen many women struggling in the same way. They may refer you to a counsellor or consider antidepressants to help you through this difficult time.

Talking therapies

When it comes to depression and anxiety, it really can be good to talk. There are a number of different talking treatments that can be carried out individually or as part of a group session. Your doctor or midwife can talk through your options, so you can access the right help for your needs. These could include:

- **Listening visits**: A specially trained health visitor can come and visit you and offer a friendly face and a supportive listening ear, without interfering or giving instructions.
- **Cognitive behavioural therapy**: CBT is a type of counselling that focuses on identifying and modifying negative ways of thinking, it can help you deal with panic attacks, anxiety, poor self-image and negative thinking. CBT is often available on the NHS and there are also self-help books and online programmes that can help you to help yourself.
- **Counselling**: A counsellor can help you talk through your feelings so you can better understand and deal with them. They can also help with setting goals and overcoming difficulties.

Medication

Medication can make a huge difference to your mental health and wellbeing. It's natural to be nervous about taking drugs in pregnancy. However, a number of antidepressants have been used safely in pregnancy for many years.

The most important thing to your baby is your health. Antidepressants can offer you the support and space to recover and feel well again. Your doctor should talk you through the risks of taking medication and the pros and cons of the treatments available to you. With help, you should see the cloud rise, so you can start to enjoy pregnancy and look forward to life with your new baby.

> *My pregnancy was planned but when the pregnancy test was actually positive it was a little shock and it felt surreal. After the initial shock, we were very happy and excited.*
>
> **~ Rachel, London**

Dr Keith says:

Once it actually dawns on you that you are pregnant, some people become apprehensive and terrified of the unknown. It's not uncommon to be more focused on getting pregnant than actually having a baby! These times can be fraught with uncertainty as the man and woman may feel differently.

Yes, pregnancy is a big deal because you have to commit to, and be responsible for, a little person for the rest of your life. The overwhelming fear of the unknown is not widely discussed in pregnancy books. Allow time and space for you and your partner to adapt to the news.

We were both excited but nervous. I particularly am anxious about the loss of control and therefore found pregnancy terrifying and stressful. I don't think anyone ever feels ready to be a parent but I knew I wanted to try. I did not think much about the lifestyle change; I was most concerned with trying to do everything in my power to protect my unborn child and offer him the best care from the start.

~ Johanna, London

Dr Keith says:

This was a first pregnancy and Johanna describes a sense of loss of control women often feel when they become pregnant for the first time. I don't think many people feel ready to become a parent. She didn't think much about the change in lifestyle; she just wanted the baby to do its best, which is generally the view of mothers to be.

To prepare yourself to be a mum, even before you start trying to conceive, it's important to chat with your partner about some of the big parenting issues, like how you'll share childcare, working versus staying home, and religious traditions. And before you start getting at loggerheads over differing opinions on subjects like circumcision, public versus private schools, or other things that are in the future, remember that you can and will change your mind about a lot of these issues as you go along. The important thing is for couples to start talking about their priorities, expectations, and fears throughout the entire process, especially before you get pregnant.

I hated being pregnant. I found it stressful to not have control, and extremely uncomfortable due to rib and back pain. Not to mention all the things you aren't allowed to do.

~ Johanna, London

Dr Keith says:

Even women who have wanted a baby for a long time, and who love that child dearly may find being pregnant a deeply unpleasant experience. Changes in your body mean it can be difficult, and more painful, to do your everyday activities and things you enjoy. As adults, we're not used to being restricted in this way. In addition to rib and back pain, women also frequently experience pain in their pelvis, and the combination of physical pain and hormonal upheaval can leave you feeling really out of sorts. Ask for help with your symptoms and get rest whenever you can. Perhaps knowing that over the centuries countless other brave mothers, perhaps even your own, have experienced the same trials and tribulations can help you deal with the challenges.

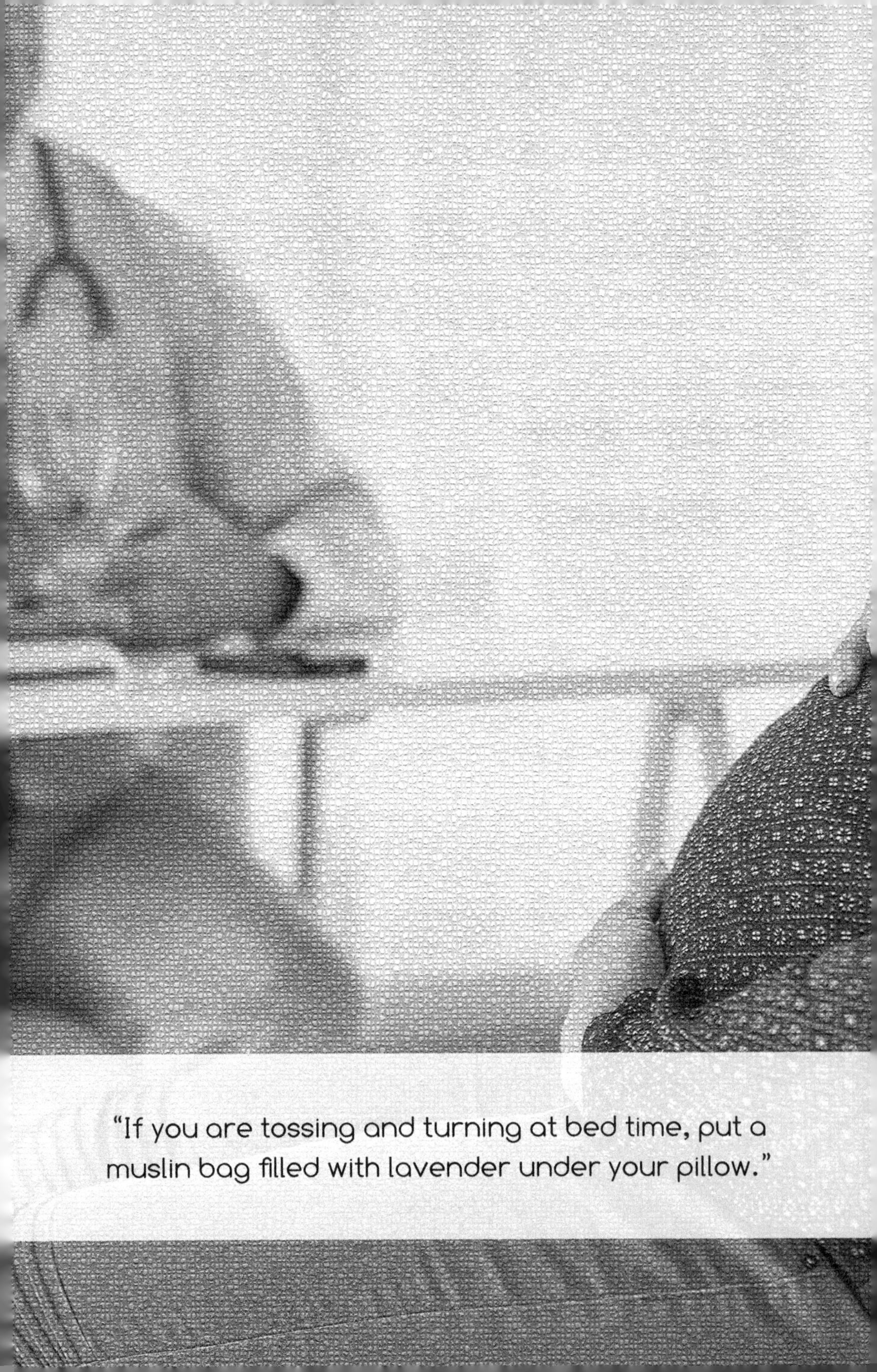

"If you are tossing and turning at bed time, put a muslin bag filled with lavender under your pillow."

17

IS IT SAFE TO USE COMPLEMENTARY THERAPIES IN PREGNANCY?

More and more expectant mums are asking me about the safe use of complementary treatments. It makes sense. Pregnancy brings with it an array of new symptoms to deal with. Nausea, insomnia, back pain, anxiety and sheer exhaustion can leave expectant mothers desperately looking for something, anything, to help them feel better. Complementary therapies can offer comfort and relief from the niggles so you can get on with enjoying your pregnancy.

An alternative approach

My patients tell me they have benefited from a whole range of treatments. Whether it's Reiki or reflexology, acupuncture or aromatherapy, the treatments can soothe your symptoms, ease anxiety and give you a much-needed energy boost.

Acupuncture in pregnancy

Acupuncture is an ancient and holistic system of healing; it treats the whole person to improve general wellbeing as well as helping soothe the individual symptoms and struggles of pregnancy.

According to traditional Chinese philosophy, our health is dependent on the body's energy (known as qi) moving smoothly through a series of channels or meridians beneath the skin. Qi is made up of equal and opposite parts—yin and yang—and when these become unbalanced, we suffer pain or become unwell.

Trained acupuncturists insert fine needles into the skin at specific points on the body, to encourage the body to heal itself and to restore its natural balance.

What can acupuncture help in pregnancy?

Acupuncture is used to treat a wide range of problems in pregnancy including back and pelvic pain and morning sickness, and for pain relief during childbirth.

Does it hurt?

For most of us, our experience of needles is limited to injections and blood tests, so many people are frightened at the idea of acupuncture. But acupuncture needles are much finer than conventional medical needles and the feeling when they're inserted is more like a tingling or a dull ache rather than the sharp bee-sting sensation of an injection.

What happens?

The acupuncturist will ask you about your symptoms, your medical history and your pregnancy. It helps if you wear loose, comfortable clothing so your therapist can easily access the acupuncture points.

The practitioner will insert fine needles into your skin at specific places, called acupuncture points. There are over 500 of these and they may be located far away from the pain or other symptom. For example, although you may suffer from headaches, needles may be inserted in your foot or hand. Needles can be inserted either for a second or two or may be left in place for thirty minutes or more, depending on the effect needed. You may feel a heaviness in your arms and legs or you may experience a pleasant relaxation.

The benefits of acupuncture frequently include more than just relief from a particular condition. Many people find it can also lead to increased energy levels, better appetite and sleep as well as an enhanced sense of overall wellbeing.

Cautions and care

I was glad to see that research in the *British Medical Journal* confirmed that acupuncture is a safe therapy when carried out by a trained professional. Serious side effects can occur after acupuncture, but the risk has been estimated as less than 1 per 10,000 treatments.

A review of the treatment in pregnancy suggested that side-effects in general were rare and usually mild. However, any therapy that has a clinical impact will also have adverse reactions. You may feel pain, have a little bleeding or bruising after treatment. Chat through any concerns with your midwife and your practitioner.

It's sensible not to plan anything strenuous after treatment because symptoms may sometimes get worse for a short time or you may feel tired and lightheaded. if you feel unwell, don't drive until your drowsiness or dizziness passes.

Reflexology in pregnancy

I don't know about you, but I find that a foot massage can help restore my wellbeing and reboot my energy. It seems I may be onto something; foot therapies were an important part of healing in many ancient cultures and are still practiced widely today.

Reflexology is much more than a foot rub. It's a natural, non-invasive method of healing. It is based on the principle that certain points on the feet and hands correspond to specific parts of the body. By applying pressure to these reflex points, a trained reflexologist can release tension, improve the blood supply and stimulate the body's natural healing processes.

Is it safe?

Many practitioners recommend avoiding reflexology during the first few months of pregnancy. There is no evidence of harm. However, at a time when you may be vulnerable to miscarriage, it can be better to stay away from all but essential treatments.

What can reflexology help in pregnancy?

Reflexology can be used simply for relaxation and health maintenance. Treatment is soothing and can help reduce feelings of stress and anxiety. Many pregnant women find reflexology beneficial for a wide range of physical symptoms and problems including tiredness, insomnia, headaches, back pain and constipation.

What happens?

Reflexology treats the body holistically. Practitioners believe that the body can be out of balance following any trauma or stress which causes the energy flow to be blocked. Reflexology treats imbalances and alleviates symptoms.

At your first session, your reflexologist will take a history of your condition and your health and explain a little about reflexology therapy. The practitioner will use pressure from their thumbs and fingers to stimulate the appropriate reflex points for you.

You may feel warmth and tingling in your feet and the rest of your body. You may also feel relaxed and drowsy; many clients fall asleep during therapy. Afterwards, you may need to use the loo more regularly (I know, even more frequently, the mind boggles). Many people feel calm and relaxed with an improvement in their symptoms.

Cautions and care

Don't take any alcohol for twenty-four hours before therapy, avoid heavy meals before treatment and drink plenty of water afterwards.

Show me the evidence

There are few reliable studies on the safety of reflexology for pregnant women, so the short answer is that we don't have a definite answer. If you feel that reflexology works for you, chat things through with your midwife and seek out a reputable and reliable therapist.

Natural remedies and pregnancy

Herbal and natural remedies, sound healthy and so harmless. But morphine comes from poppies, aspirin is extracted from willow bark and the powerful heart drug digoxin is made from foxgloves. Medications that come from nature can be powerful and effective but they are not without problems and side-effects.

I don't want to scare you. Natural medicines can offer relief from the discomforts of pregnancy. But do your research first, see a qualified practitioner, don't take anything that isn't clearly labelled and chat with your midwife or doctor before starting a course of treatment.

Herbal medicine

Herbal remedies in pregnancy have been handed down from grandmother to mother, to daughter. Ginger, raspberry leaf tea, chamomile and peppermint have been used for centuries to ease discomfort, nausea and insomnia. They really have stood the test of time and for many treatments, research is confirming what your great granny already knew—they can really work.

But, of course, if a substance is powerful enough to make a difference to your symptoms, it can also be powerful enough to cause side-effects and interfere with prescribed medication. You need to be careful and follow the advice of a qualified medical herbalist or a trained midwife.

Herbal helpers

- **Raspberry leaf tea**: Sipping a daily cuppa from 32 weeks can help tone and strengthen the womb, so you have a shorter, smoother labour.
- **Ginger**: Whether it's brewed as a tea or munched as a biscuit, ginger may help ease nausea and morning sickness.
- **Peppermint**: Try peppermint tea, or a little extract to beat bloating and ban indigestion.
- **Chamomile**: Are you tossing, turning and desperately trying to sleep? Swap your English Breakfast for a cup of chamomile to soothe you to sleep and calm your nerves.

It worked for me

I had terrible wind and bloating in pregnancy but didn't want to take any drugs. My midwife suggested peppermint tea, which was totally delicious and did the business for my bowels too. Any time my tummy feels uncomfortable or uneasy, it's my go-to remedy.

~ Louise, York

Chinese herbal medicine

Chinese herbal medicine is an ancient method of healing that harnesses the special properties of plants to treat illness and maintain good health. It is believed to work holistically to correct the body's imbalances rather than to treat individual symptoms. There is also an emphasis on managing our lifestyles to prevent disease before it occurs. When the body is in balance, our natural healing processes are stimulated and we can have a happier and healthier pregnancy.

What happens?

At the first consultation, the practitioner will ask you about your symptoms, your pregnancy and your medical history. They will also do a physical examination, taking your pulse and inspecting your tongue. The practitioner may then give you advice about your diet, lifestyle and exercise and make up a prescription.

The herbs may come in different forms: A tincture, which is a concentrated solution of herbs in water and alcohol, tablets, ointment and 'raw herbs', which have to be boiled in water and drunk as a tea. You will be asked to return for a follow up appointment, so it's useful to take note of any changes in your health and symptoms,

Cautions and care

Herbal medicines are like other medications and should be used with extreme care. They can interact with other drugs and some are not safe in pregnancy. It is essential to use a reputable, qualified and experienced Chinese Herbal Practitioner. Tell them you are pregnant, if you are on prescribed medication, and also talk through any treatments with your GP or midwife.

Poorly made or labelled medicines can be a health risk. The Medical Toxicology Unit at Guy's and St Thomas' NHS Trust suggests you ask for a list of the ingredients in any herbal product you buy or are given, so if there are any side effects, the causal ingredient can be identified.

Reiki in pregnancy

Reiki is an alternative method of healing developed in Japan. The word Reiki can be translated as 'universal life energy'. An experienced Reiki practitioner is able to recognise and use this invisible energy. Therapists believe they can stimulate the body's natural healing processes and the flow of this life force throughout the body.

What can Reiki help?

Reiki is used for a wide range of conditions, including physical problems, and to relieve mental and emotional distress. In pregnancy, it can encourage relaxation and help you fall asleep. It is also thought to ease back and pelvic girdle pain and may provide some relief from nausea and morning sickness.

Regular treatment may help you have a smoother and less stressful labour and delivery. The Reiki skills you learn could be useful after the birth too, to keep your baby calm and comfortable.

What happens?

There are many variations of Reiki. It's a healing process that works at bringing us into balance and reinforcing the body's natural ability to heal itself, physically, mentally, emotionally and spiritually. It's not a cure but is a natural form of healing that can be used to support and enhance other forms of treatment, both medical and complementary.

Your Reiki treatment should take place in a peaceful and relaxing environment. Although you will need to remove your coat and shoes, it's not necessary to take off any other clothing. The practitioner will take your medical history and find out more about your pregnancy and any problems you're hoping to address.

The practitioner gently places their hands non-intrusively, on or near the body. There is no massage or manipulation and the whole person is treated rather than specific symptoms.

You may feel a flow of energy, mild tingling, warmth, coolness or nothing at all. At times, you may spontaneously release emotion as your energy rebalances. Crying can be a natural and healthy part of the therapy.

Cautions and care

It is advisable to rest after a Reiki treatment and drink lots of water. Treatment is generally thought to be safe and can be used alongside conventional medical treatments. However, you should tell your doctor or and midwife if you are having any other complementary or conventional medical treatments.

Show me the evidence

The research evidence on whether Reiki actually works is rather mixed, although it does appear to be a safe therapy. There may be some benefit when it is used to alleviate pain and anxiety but more studies are definitely needed. If you feel Reiki benefits you, chat to your midwife and make sure you see a reputable Reiki master who will assess you properly and treat you with care.

Are they safe?

Whether you're planning acupuncture for pain, or a herbal blend to knock you out at bedtime, it's important to check with your doctor or midwife before starting any form of alternative treatment.

Many complementary therapies are still unregulated, so it can be difficult to find the right practitioner. However, there are wonderful, experienced and professional therapists out there. Do your research and ask family, friends and your midwife for their recommendations. Remember to choose a practitioner who's trained, registered, insured and, vitally, experienced at treating pregnant women.

18

IS BABY BRAIN A MYTH?

Pregnancy affects your whole body from the top of your head to the tip of your toes, so it can be no surprise that it will have an impact on your brain. Your mood, your thoughts and even your dreams can be affected.

Pregnant women often joke with me their brains have turned to mush. They walk into the kitchen and forget what they've come for, are less able to focus at work or feel generally emotional instead of incisive. But is there a physiological reason for this, or is it the natural result of the exhaustion of juggling the demands of work and home as well as nurturing a new life? Does baby brain really exist?

Normal or not?

As many as four in five women say they go into a sort of pregnancy fog. They may become forgetful, their mind feels less sharp and they find they are a little over sensitive and less able to concentrate. But are they simply attributing totally normal experiences to pregnancy? Let's face it, we all misplace our phones or lose our train of thought every now and again. It could be that our cultural expectations mean that as soon as the thin blue line appears on the pregnancy test, it is blamed for every little failure and foible.

Brain changes

The truth is that the research into this subject is mixed. Some studies suggest that the hormonal surge of pregnancy may prepare your brain for the many challenges of maternity, helping you stay calm and become in tune with your baby's needs. Researchers at the University of London examined the brains of pregnant women and found increased activity in the area that affects emotions. Pregnant women tended to use the right side of the brain more when they were processing emotions. The researchers suggested that this could be a natural adaptation to help prepare them to bond with their babies. The change in brain activity seemed to help women recognise emotions in others. This increased emotional intelligence may come at the expense of other cognitive functions, so women think differently rather than less.

More recent research showed no significant difference between the memories and mental skills of women who were pregnant compared to those who weren't. This was despite the fact that the pregnant women did complain of significantly greater difficulties, so what's going on?

Dr Keith says:

A Canadian study in 2011 caught my eye. They found that pregnant women did not display any problems at all in lab-based cognitive tests. However, they were significantly more likely to forget to phone the lab on time or to return their questionnaires. So it could be that the quiet lab environment enabled them to focus, whereas the distractions and competing demands of normal life can make things more tricky.

> *I got super forgetful in pregnancy. Like I would set something down and never find it again or get distracted from tasks easily. I think a lot of it was to do with the fact I wanted to be organised and get everything ready. I suppose trying to juggle so many balls at one time made my brain go silly!*
>
> **~ Lindsey, Kilkeel**

Practical matters

Whatever the reason for your mental changes, you can help yourself cut through the pregnancy fog.

- Make sure you rest and relax, get plenty of sleep and schedule pauses into your day. Don't think of it as laziness. By recharging your batteries you can continue performing to the best of your ability.
- Trigger your memory: it can help to make lists, set phone reminders and use the same storage place for your keys, purse and mobile, so you minimise daily stresses and strains.
- Embrace your new talents, your pregnancy may have helped you become more intuitive and responsive to the needs of others.

Above all, be kind to yourself. We all make mistakes. If you forget something, don't beat yourself up. Remember that your body is doing the extraordinary job of growing a whole new being, so look after it, nurture it and above all, cut it some slack if it occasionally lets you down!

Pregnancy dreams

Even when you're sleeping, your body will still be hard at work building your baby, and you may find your brain will be equally active. Pregnancy definitely stimulates some vivid and varied dreams.

Why do we dream?

Dreams reflect your own emotional state, but in a distorted and different way. They're a way for your mind to process your thoughts and experiences.

A dreamy pregnancy?

With all the excitement, stress and life change pregnancy brings, it's little wonder that your dreams are intense. The raised levels of the hormone progesterone can increase the emotional rollercoaster.

Lots of people tell me they have never really dreamed before pregnancy. But that's because dreams typically happen during the rapid-eye movement (REM) stage of sleep. It's when the brain is active and firing—if you pull back an eyelid it will show that your eyes are continually moving during this stage. If you wake up a while after this phase, you may not remember what you have dreamed. But in pregnancy, you're up and down all the time. You may need a wee, your leg cramps, you get a numb hand from carpal tunnel syndrome—long unbroken sleeps are pretty rare. This means that the chances of waking up with your mind full of memories of a recent dream are much greater.

Will it affect my baby?

The good news is that your baby is in your womb, not your brain. No matter what scary or salacious things your mind has been conjuring up, your unborn child will be blissfully unaware. Whether you're active, snoozing or dreaming, your baby will still be able to rest and wriggle to their heart's content.

What do my dreams mean?

Dream doctors believe that your pregnancy dreams reflect your current experiences and your feelings about the birth. So, if you dream you left your baby in the supermarket, maybe you're feeling worried you won't be a good mum. Picturing an ill, deformed or even inhuman baby can reflect your understandable stress and anxiety about your baby's health.

That's not my child

Lots of women dream they have given birth to an animal or an alien. Don't panic, it has nothing to do with reality. It can be down to simple anxiety and the ET like appearance of your baby on the scan. Or it could be a way of your mind practising for the real thing. A puppy or a kitten are familiar and unthreatening and this sort of visualisation can help your subconscious rehearse for the future.

I'm not worthy

You've left your baby on the bus, the pram is running off down the hill and you can't catch it or you've dropped your baby from your arms. There are a million ways that your mind can represent your fears about not being a good enough mum.

I can't get out

Being enclosed in a small room or a cupboard, or feeling stuck and unable to move, can be a recurring dream. It may reflect the new sense of responsibility you feel and perhaps worry about being tied down.

Overindulgence

Gorging on cakes, binging on booze or lighting up a cigarette can make you wake up feeling guilty. But don't stress. The tricks of your imagination won't harm your baby. It's common when you've given something up, or you're eating more healthily, for your lifestyle changes to occupy your waking and sleeping thoughts for a while. With time, these dreams should fade.

Naked charm

You're nude in the supermarket, or chairing an important meeting in your underwear. Naked dreams really are a nightmare. They often signify insecurity, which with all the changes going on in your life, wouldn't be too surprising.

Cheats between the sheets

Have you ever woken up furious with your partner because they had an affair in your dreams? Cheating dreams can feel disturbingly real, and even though you KNOW it didn't really happen, it can be tricky to totally forgive them!

Pregnancy dramatically changes your body, which can make some women feel unattractive and insecure. This vulnerability can be reflected in dreams about infidelity and betrayal.

Water, water everywhere

Dreams about swimming, waterfalls and standing in the sea are common throughout pregnancy. It could be a way of connecting with your unborn child who's also splashing around in water within your womb. Sometimes the water imagery can be less pleasant, though, with drowning or struggling for air being a frequent dream. This could be because you are feeling overwhelmed with the experience of pregnancy and the upcoming birth.

Blasts from the past

At a time when new life is about to be created, many women find that their nightly thoughts are filled with lost friends and family members. This feeling can be wonderful, rather than macabre, with time spent with grandparents who have passed away. You may feel a renewed sense of loss in the morning, but experts believe that these dreams are your mind's way of processing loss and linking past generations with the new generation to come.

Steamy stuff

Pregnancy can sometimes put you off intercourse, but that doesn't mean your mind has given up on sexy stuff. Lots of expectant mums have strange sexual dreams that can make Fifty Shades of Grey seem tame. Sex in public, strange partners, a gender you've never found attractive, anything and everything can be dreamed up. It's probably down to those hormones again. It's particularly common in the early weeks, and could be because there's increased blood flow to your breasts and pelvis, meaning they're more easily stimulated, so you get turned-on. It has such an effect that lots of women can orgasm spontaneously in their sleep. Even more reason to schedule a cheeky nap into your day!

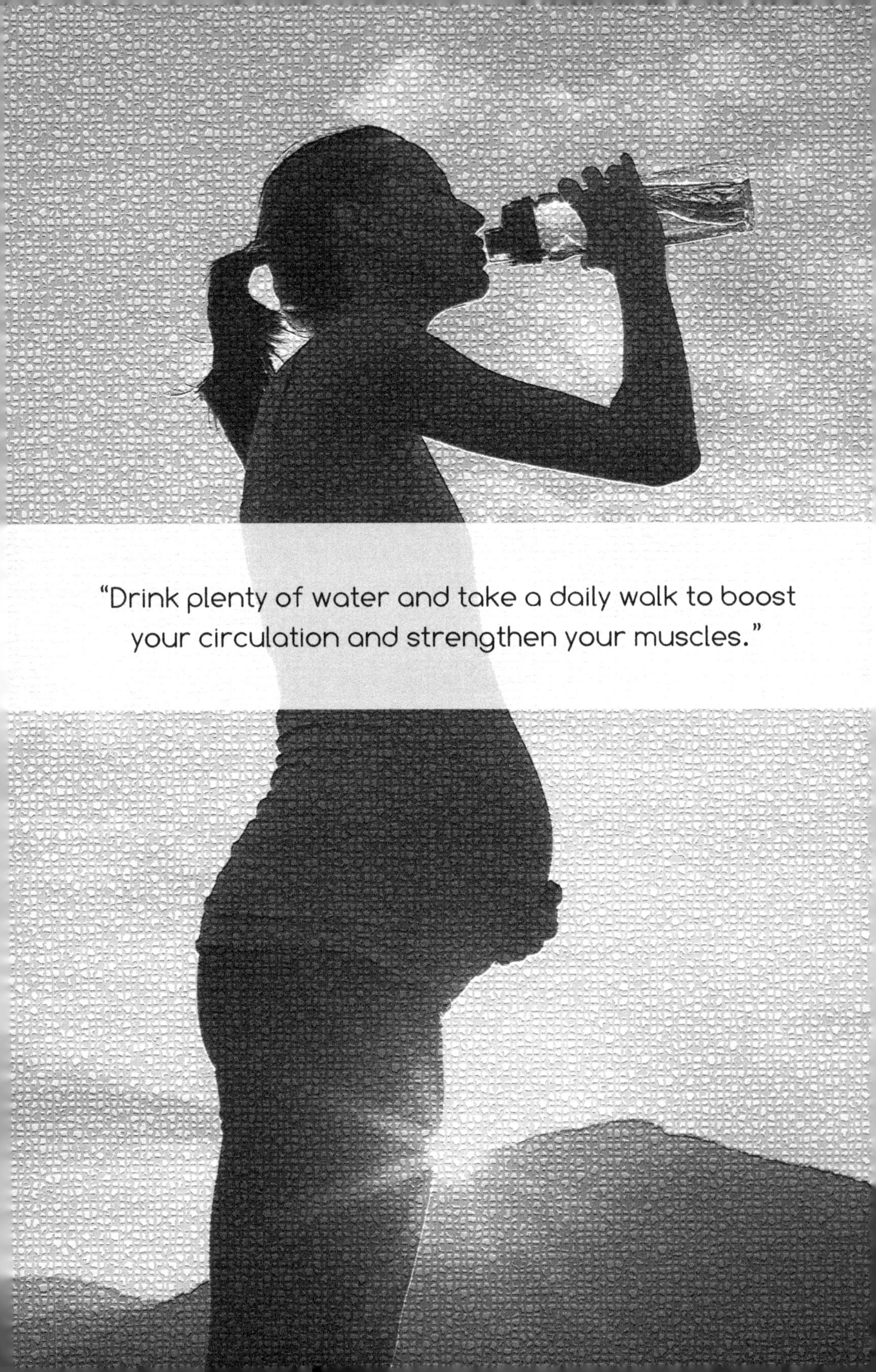
"Drink plenty of water and take a daily walk to boost your circulation and strengthen your muscles."

19

WHAT CAN I DO ABOUT VARICOSE VEINS?

If you thought that varicose veins only affected old ladies, think again. As many as two in five pregnant women develop these blue, swollen and gnarled veins in pregnancy. They tend to appear in the legs, in the back passage as piles and sometimes in the vulva too. Did someone say pregnancy was glamorous?

They're caused by your growing womb pressing against the veins in the pelvis, combined with the hormones relaxing the walls of your veins and the extra blood circulating.

Sadly, they seem to get worse with each pregnancy, so I wouldn't advise definitive treatment until you have completed your family!

Why me?

Varicose veins tend to run in families, so check-out your mum's legs if you want to see if you're at risk. They're also more likely to appear if you gain a lot of weight during pregnancy, so protect yourself by staying active, being sensible and not eating for two.

What can I do?

When it comes to varicose veins, it's not just a matter of vanity. As well as being unsightly they can also be painful and problematic. Even though you can't get rid of them, you can improve your symptoms:

- Take a daily walk to boost your circulation and strengthen your leg muscles.
- Don't cross your legs when you're sitting down. It can restrict blood flow and make you more likely to develop spider or thread veins.
- Rest and put your feet up whenever you can and remember to rotate your ankles every now and again to keep the blood flowing.
- Wear elasticated support tights to stop the veins filling up and prevent ugly bulging as well as any aching.
- An apple a day. A healthy balanced diet is important. If you're worried about varicose veins, boost your vitamin C levels to help keep the connective tissues in the veins healthy.

> *I had varicose veins in both my pregnancies. I found that keeping support tights under my pillow and putting them on before I got out of bed was the best way of stopping them aching during the day.*
>
> **~ Sally, Newcastle**

The good news is that varicose veins usually disappear within a few months of the birth. The bad news is that they're likely to pop right back out again in future pregnancies, so don't chuck out that support hose yet.

Piles in pregnancy

People snigger about their 'Farmer Giles', but for lots of women in pregnancy, they're no laughing matter. Piles (or haemorrhoids) are like varicose veins in the back passage. And one thing I can tell you for sure is that they've got nothing to do with sitting on cold, stone walls. They're caused by the womb pressing on the pelvic veins and are made worse by pushing in labour, constipation and straining to go to the loo.

You'll know you have them if you see bright red blood splashing around the pan when you have a poo, if your anus is sore, uncomfortable or itchy or if you notice something coming down when you open your bowels.

Preventing piles

You can fight piles by avoiding constipation and ensuring you don't strain to pass a motion. Tuck into a high fibre diet with loads of fresh fruit and veggies, pulses, beans and wholegrains. Drink plenty of fluid to keep things soft. Sip water, fresh fruit or prune juice throughout the day. If you're still constipated, see your healthcare team for stool softeners, fibre supplements or a gentle laxative to get everything moving again.

What should I do?

If you notice a small haemorrhoid, you can push it back in gently using lubricating jelly and a clean finger. An ice compress or haemorrhoid cream will relieve pain and ease any itching.

The good news is that although haemorrhoids can be horribly uncomfortable, they usually disappear soon after the birth and rarely cause any serious problems. So it's safe to fill up on fibre and fluid and wait. However, if you are suffering increasing pain and bleeding, it's essential to see your doctor for a check-up.

Mum's conundrum

I keep reading that I shouldn't put on too much weight in pregnancy. All the books and websites say that too much could give me piles and varicose veins and diabetes but no one will give me a normal healthy figure for weight gain. It's so frustrating. How much is too much?

~ Ellie, Birmingham

Dr Keith says:

Most women gain some weight in pregnancy. Let's face it, the extra blood, breast tissue and fluid, not to mention the baby, placenta and amniotic fluid, mean that some extra kilos are almost inevitable. Indeed, a healthy weight gain can protect against having a low birth weight baby with the associated health risks.

But what is a healthy weight gain? Like you, lots of women ask me for precise figures. But the truth is that there is little good research on this subject. Pregnancy weight gain varies hugely between individuals, with the average falling between ten and twelve and a half kilos, or between twenty-two and twenty-eight pounds.

How much is too much?

I think the 'right' amount of weight for each individual depends on their height, their build and crucially their weight before they got pregnant. Women who are obese or overweight can safely gain less weight, whereas those who have a low BMI before conception may need to put on a few more pounds to ensure the health and wellbeing of their baby.

But although a certain amount of weight gain can be healthy, too much definitely isn't. It's not just that it's difficult to shed the excess weight after the birth. Women who pile on the pounds also have a higher risk of complications including gestational diabetes, miscarriage, pre-eclampsia, blood clots and even maternal death. And it's not just the mother's health that is hit. A baby born to an obese mother is at higher risk of stillbirth, congenital abnormalities and obesity in the future. Weight gain is about much more than vanity and fitting back into those pre-pregnancy jeans.

What makes up the 'baby' weight?

It can be a nasty surprise after the birth when your body doesn't shrink back to its pre-pregnancy state. How much is down to baby and how much is extra padding? Well, at birth your baby weighs on average 3.3 kilos, the placenta comes in at 0.7 of a kilo and the amniotic fluid will make up another 0.8 of a kilo of the extra weight you are carrying. When the baby is delivered you'll have shed 4.8 eight kilos or between ten and eleven pounds. That doesn't sound much does it?

Much of the rest of the excess weight is down to changes in your own body, this will naturally gradually subside over the postnatal period. Your stronger, larger womb could account for up to a kilo, the increased blood volume can weigh in at 1.2 kilos and body fluid can also make up 1.2 kilos. And what about your magnificent, enlarged breasts? Well they can push the scales another half a kilogram to the right. That's another 3.9 kilos or eight and a half pounds.

Any weight over and above this is body fat. But don't panic or get despondent; some fat is absolutely essential. Your body stores it up to prepare you for the rigours of breastfeeding. It's important to have laid down an extra three or four kilos, especially if you were underweight before pregnancy, so you have the necessary reserves available to allow your body to cope with the energy demands of feeding your new baby.

Dieting to lose weight during pregnancy is not recommended, unless under the close supervision of an expert medical team. Cutting down on essential food may mean that there's simply not enough energy and micronutrients for the healthy growth and development of your unborn child. However, some research in the British Medical Journal caught my eye. Doctors carefully managed the weight of women who had gained too much in pregnancy.

Dr Daghni Rajasingam, a spokesperson for the Royal College of Obstetricians and Gynaecologists said:

'There is a growing body of research to suggest that weight management in pregnancy for women who put on excessive weight can be beneficial and reduce the risk of complications. This paper shows that for some women, managing weight gain is safe.

However, it is important to note that the ideal time for losing weight for obese and overweight women is before conception. A healthy diet and exercise before, during and after pregnancy is recommended'

I'd echo this. It's better to optimise your fitness and get to a healthy BMI before pregnancy, so during pregnancy, you can focus on nourishing your body and your baby.

20

CAN I PROTECT MYSELF AGAINST GESTATIONAL DIABETES?

More and more women are asking me this question. It's probably a reflection of the increasing awareness of the condition, which can only be a good thing.

What is gestational diabetes?

Gestational diabetes is a type of diabetes that can develop in pregnancy. Blood sugar levels go up because the body isn't producing enough insulin for its increasing needs. Insulin is the hormone released when we eat. It works to allow the body's muscles and tissues to use glucose for energy and safely store any excess.

Who is affected?

As many as one in twenty pregnant women in the UK will develop gestational diabetes, and the numbers appear to be increasing. Sometimes, developing diabetes can be a matter of bad luck. However, there are a number of factors that can put you at increased risk.

- **A history of gestational diabetes**: If you became diabetic during a previous pregnancy, you are likely to develop it in subsequent pregnancies.
- **Big baby**: If you have previously had a baby who weighed more than ten pounds at birth, you have an increased risk of gestational diabetes when you become pregnant again.
- **Obesity**: Being overweight can increase your risk of type 2 diabetes and of developing gestational diabetes in pregnancy. So you should be particularly careful if you have a BMI over 30.
- **Family history**: A tendency towards diabetes can run in some families. You are more at risk if a close relative has had gestational or type 2 diabetes.
- **Ethnicity**: Women from Afro-Caribbean, South Asian or Middle Eastern backgrounds are more likely to develop diabetes in pregnancy.

A quick glance at that list will show you that there are lots of things you can't change. No one can alter their medical history, their genetic heritage or their ethnicity. But we can all work to get to a healthy BMI, which will decrease the risk of developing diabetes in pregnancy. It also helps to eat a healthy balanced diet, not to gain too much weight in pregnancy and to stay active to protect yourself against developing the condition.

> *I didn't meet any of the stereotypes or categories that put me at risk of diabetes but I still developed it. Work was so stressful for me, there were possible redundancies and the company was running into major cash-flow problems, as it was a charity. I think the stress took its toll on my body and it put my blood sugars up and I had to go to the diabetes clinic every week from thirty weeks!*
>
> **~ Suzie, Lisburn**

Dr Keith says:

Lots of women get stressed out in pregnancy but too much worry can boost the body's levels of the hormone cortisol. Cortisol has a vital role in raising plasma glucose levels at times of stress, so the body has the energy it needs to face attacks from injury, illness or infection. This was great when we were cavemen and women fighting sabre-toothed tigers—but less ideal in modern lives when stress can be psychological and constant.

Too much cortisol for too long can be damaging. So in some women, maybe with other risk factors, stress could make developing gestational diabetes a little more likely. Don't panic, though, there's lots you can do to help yourself: regular exercise, taking time out to rest and relax, mindfulness meditation and simply learning to say no to impossible demands and being kind to yourself can be brilliant stress busters, allowing you to stay calm and enjoy your pregnancy.

How will I know?

Gestational diabetes usually develops in the third trimester, often between 24 and 28 weeks. The classic signs of diabetes include feeling exhausted, being constantly thirsty and spending all day on the loo. But that sounds like the normal symptoms of pregnancy, doesn't it?

The good news is that all pregnant women in the UK who are thought to be at risk will be offered a test to screen for gestational diabetes and your urine will be checked for glucose at every antenatal appointment. If you have one of these risk factors, your doctor may send you for a screening test before 16 weeks. Your midwife may also identify that you're developing diabetes during your antenatal appointments. When the blood sugar levels rise, some leaks out into the urine so it can be picked up with dipsticks.

In my experience, we are becoming more efficient at picking up gestational diabetes. Many are diagnosed with the condition before they become unwell or notice any significant symptoms. But don't be complacent; many women have no risk factors. If you're feeling tired, thirsty and unwell, don't dismiss your symptoms. Talk to your midwife or doctor.

Protecting yourself from gestational diabetes

Your doctor and midwife will make a note of any risk factors and keep a close eye on you to ensure you and your baby remain well. However, it is also sensible to look after your own wellbeing, eat a healthy balanced diet and seek help if you feel unwell.

Lots of health professionals will be supporting and guiding you throughout your pregnancy, but ultimately you are in charge of your body. By taking control of your lifestyle you can help yourself stay healthy, decrease the danger of diabetes and protect your developing baby.

Preconception planning

The best time to get to a healthy BMI is before pregnancy starts. Choosing a healthy nutritious diet will increase your fertility, nourish your body and help you get to an optimum BMI for pregnancy of between 20 and 25. If you're a little heavy, especially if your BMI is above 30, see your doctor for support to lose weight.

Eat well

A healthy diet in pregnancy can provide the micronutrients your developing baby needs and prevent you piling on the pounds. Alex Davies, head of prevention for the National Charity Partnership, said that the eating for two myth was unhelpful:

Eating healthily and consuming healthy portion sizes are important before, during and after pregnancy to increase the chances of conceiving naturally, reduce the risk of pregnancy and birth-related complications and stave off health problems like type 2 diabetes and heart and circulatory disease in the long-term.

So cut back on sugar, white bread, cakes and cookies. Instead tuck into loads of fresh fruit and vegetables, lean meat, fish, pulses, dairy and legumes. Replace wholegrains for white carbs and your sugars and your mood will both be more stable. You'll probably find you're less hungry, too. What's not to like?

An active life

Exercising before conception and during pregnancy can make you happier, healthier and fit for the demands of labour. But it won't just benefit your wellbeing, it will also help ensure you build a healthy baby. Regular activity can reduce weight gain and may decrease your risk of gestational diabetes. If you do develop the condition, activity can decrease your blood glucose and may prevent you needing to take medication or insulin. That's worth getting off the sofa for, isn't it?

The fitness factor

When you work your body, your cells use up the glucose in your bloodstream. If you're struggling to keep your sugar levels down with careful control of your diet, increasing your activity levels can give them a nudge in the right direction.

The good news is that to get results you don't have to run a marathon, pump iron or go for the burn. Even modest increases in your level of physical activity will make a difference. Try walking for half an hour every day, taking the stairs instead of the lift, swimming or even hitting the dance floor to increase the energy you burn and boost your level of fitness.

Ban the baddies

If you develop gestational diabetes, there is an increase in the likelihood of complications in your pregnancy, so it's a good idea to get rid of any other risk factors by kicking any bad habits. Make sure you quit alcohol and cigarettes to give your baby the best chance of a healthy life.

What will happen if you develop gestational diabetes?

When you are already coping with the physical and emotional strains of pregnancy, discovering you have gestational diabetes can be terrifying. But there's no need to panic. Your team will have lots of experience in dealing with diabetes and can help you control your sugar levels and stay healthy. With support, information, the right treatment and lifestyle changes, you can remain well and protect your unborn child.

Antenatal care

It's important to take gestational diabetes seriously; high sugar levels can put your health at risk and affect the development of your baby. Uncontrolled diabetes is associated with higher levels of Caesarean section, difficult births, big babies and, sadly, increased rates of late pregnancy loss.

That sounds scary, but the good news is that you and your antenatal care team can work together to control your sugars and protect your health as well as that of your baby.

Your antenatal care team will give you blood sugar targets and a monitor so you can keep your glucose levels at the optimum level for you and your baby.

For many people, their diabetes can be controlled with diet and exercise alone. That doesn't mean weight loss. Instead, you should focus on a healthy balanced diet, cutting back on refined carbs and sugars. Tuck into lots of veggies, some fruit, plenty of fish, pulses and wholegrains and stay away from sugary stuff, processed and fast foods, which are often high in calories and low in nutrients.

It's not a good idea to embark on a rigorous exercise regime if you're not used to it. Instead try to live an active life, with plenty of long walks and swims to burn off extra energy. Sometimes medication is also needed to get your glucose levels down. This may be tablets or sometimes insulin may need to be injected to achieve the best control.

Diabetes in labour

It's a good idea to give birth in hospital so there will be plenty of assistance and medical back-up if there are any problems during the birth or afterwards. Your blood glucose levels will be carefully monitored and you may need a drip to keep things stable if they are becoming too high or too low.

Your baby will need to be fed regularly to keep their blood sugar levels stable. Your midwife should support you to do the first feed within half an hour of the birth and every two to three hours after that. They will also check their glucose levels with a pinprick, in the same way as you have been monitoring yours. At least twenty-four hours of close monitoring will be needed to check for any medical problems and make sure that breastfeeding is established or your baby is bottle-feeding well and their blood glucose is stable.

Postnatal care

Usually, your body's insulin needs will drop dramatically immediately after the birth, so any medication will be stopped to ensure your sugars don't become dangerously low. Your levels will be checked on discharge and again at your six-week check. However, it's essential to see your doctor immediately if any symptoms are returning, because sometimes pregnancy can reveal underlying diabetes.

What does it mean for the future?

After having gestational diabetes, you are at increased risk of developing type 2 diabetes in the future as well as having gestational diabetes in future pregnancies. But this tendency doesn't have to be your destiny. You can make changes to help protect yourself. Arrange an annual blood glucose test with your GP to keep an eye on things. Try to lose weight to reach a healthy BMI, eat a balanced diet and exercise regularly. By taking control of your own weight, fitness and wellbeing, you can keep yourself healthy and well for future pregnancies and future life.

21

I'M SO WILD AND WINDY. HOW CAN PREGNANCY AFFECT DIGESTION?

When you look at Instagram images of gently undulating bumps and glowing mums-to-be, it can seem that everyone else is sailing through pregnancy with effortless ease. But pregnancy can do some weird, wacky and downright embarrassing things to your body. So if you're belching, bunged up or making some strange noises, don't worry, you're not alone!

Constipation in pregnancy

Sickness, the incessant need to wee and having bunged up bowels can mean it feels like you spend most of your pregnancy in the loo. I'm probably repeating myself, but in case you're only reading this section, I will reiterate that constipation is a common problem, affecting around half of pregnant women. It leaves lots of people writhing with discomfort and frustration. Fortunately, there's lots you can do to get things moving again and keep your bowels relaxed and regular.

Why me?

The hormone progesterone tends to make the bowel work a little slower in pregnancy, which can predispose to constipation. Iron supplements, dehydration due to vomiting and pressure from the growing baby can make the problem worse. The good news is we know a few tricks to help you combat constipation:

What can I do?

- **Eat a high fibre diet** with loads of fresh fruit and vegetables, pulses, beans and wholegrains. Dried apricots, prunes and raisins pack a fibre punch and will boost your iron.
- **Drink up.** Dehydration will bung you up. Slurp down plenty of water and other fluids throughout the day. A glass of prune juice, warm water with lemon or a hot cup of tea are tricks mums tell me have worked to help them get things going.
- **Ask your doctor if you're taking supplements.** Iron tablets can cause constipation. Choose iron rich foods to prevent anaemia and see your GP for a different formulation or a lower dose if you're struggling to cope.
- **Keep moving.** Regular exercise can ease constipation and make you fitter. Walking, swimming or yoga can stop that sluggish feeling in your body and your bowels.
- **Don't strain.** If it won't come, don't force it. You'll put yourself at risk of piles and anal tears. Instead, up your fibre and fluids and see your doctor for softeners or suppositories.
- **Don't miss the moment.** Listen to your body. When the urge comes, head straight to the loo.

Remember, you don't have to suffer alone. If the fibre, fluid and fitness is not working, it's time to see your doctor. Don't be embarrassed, it's a common pregnancy problem and we really can help. Medications to boost your fibre, soften your stools or act as a gentle laxative can help loosen things up and soothe your discomfort so you have one less thing to worry about.

Diarrhoea in pregnancy

While most pregnant women tell me their bowels become sluggish in pregnancy, some find that their intestines head in the opposite direction. If you're struggling with frequent loose or runny motions, it's more likely to be due to something unrelated to pregnancy, or if you're reaching term, it could be an exciting indication that your baby is finally on their way.

- **New diet, new diarrhoea**: Lots of women change their diets in pregnancy. If you've been inspired by my guides to healthy eating you may be tucking into lots of fresh fruit and veggies and plenty of wholegrains. That's fantastic, but it may take your guts a little while to adapt to the extra fibre passing through.
- **Supplements**: Some women find that certain multivitamin or supplement formulations can upset their tummies. If you suspect yours is loosening things up, try a different brand.
- **Bugs and bacteria**: Don't assume that the symptoms you develop are down to pregnancy. The normal infections that can strike us all can also affect pregnant women. Food poisoning, tummy bugs, parasites and viruses can cause diarrhoea whether you're pregnant or not.
- **Labour**: Late on in pregnancy, loose bowel movements together with a little nausea or vomiting, can be an early signal that you're going into labour.

What should I do?

The most important thing for your baby's wellbeing is your own health. Diarrhoea isn't just a pain in the butt, it can lead to dehydration, which can put you at risk of early labour. Take it seriously and look after yourself.

A few loose stools are unlikely to be a concern, but if you're going more than three times a day, if there's blood or mucous or you're feeling feverish or unwell, see your doctor urgently.

Rehydrate: Keep sipping fluids to hydrate your body. Avoid sugary drinks and juices which can make symptoms worse. Instead, try clear water or electrolyte-rich sports drinks.

Healthy bacteria: Our guts are home to a mind-boggling five hundred million bacteria that help us maintain a healthy digestion and break down the fibre in our food. Having the right balance between good and bad bacteria is vital for our health and wellbeing. Boost your good bacteria by enjoying live yoghurt as a snack.

Be a BRAT: Choose foods that are gentle on the bowel to give your system a rest. The BRAT diet of **b**ananas, **r**ice, **a**pplesauce and **t**oast can help provide sustenance and energy while you recover. Try adding lean meats for protein and clear soups as you can manage them. It's a good idea to stay away from heavy, fried and fatty foods and anything too spicy until you're feeling much better.

Indigestion and heartburn in pregnancy

Indigestion and heartburn can unsettle your stomach and set your gullet on fire from as early as six weeks into the pregnancy until the day of delivery. It affects up to eight out of ten expectant mums and it's down to those pregnancy hormones and the growing baby inside you.

Early on, progesterone (the hormone that stops womb contractions until the time of labour) slows the passage of food and decreases the speed at which your stomach empties. This can leave you feeling bloated, nauseous and with a tendency to burp at the wrong moments! The hormones also relax the valve at the stomach entrance, so acid contents can flow back up the oesophagus causing a burning sensation in the centre of the chest. This effect gets worse whenever gravity lends a helping hand, so be careful when you're in bed, lying flat or bending over.

In the last trimester, you may find yourself burping and belching like a corpulent Dickensian character. As well as your pregnancy hormones making your stomach contents flow back up the gullet, the growing bump pushes up against the stomach so you feel bloated, full and flatulent.

How can I help?

- **Little and often**: Eating small frequent meals will ensure you get the nutrients you need without overfilling your stomach.
- **Bland is best**: Stay away from spicy and fried foods, which may worsen symptoms.
- **Eat early**: Don't eat within three hours of going to bed to allow your food to digest and decrease night-time discomfort.
- **Bin bad habits**: If you haven't already stopped smoking and drinking alcohol in pregnancy, now's the time. Booze and fags can inflame your stomach and increase pain, plus quitting them is better for your baby. It's a win, win situation.
- **Avoid triggers**: Coffee, cola, tea, chocolate and even bending over can bring on the burn. Keep an eye on what triggers you and try to cut those things out.
- **Sleep safely**: Get a good night's sleep by propping yourself up with pillows, or by raising the head end of the mattress with some chunky books. Keep a glass of milk or some dry biscuits or crackers to hand to settle your stomach.
- **Beat the burn**: Some over the counter antacids like Settlers, Rennies or Gaviscon are safe if used according to instructions,

in pregnancy. See your pharmacist or talk to your midwife for advice.

Usually, changes to your diet and lifestyle can help calm indigestion and keep you comfortable through pregnancy. However, if your indigestion is severe and you're struggling to eat or sleep, see your doctor. Your GP may suggest using medication to block the acid and quell the fire in your stomach.

I had terrible problems with constipation when I took iron tablets in my first pregnancy. This time I ate loads of watercress and dried apricots and it's worked a treat—I'm not anaemic and I've had no constipation either.

~ Vicky, Harrogate

22

IS IT SAFE TO EAT FOR TWO?

So many women ask me this question that I was not surprised to discover that a recent survey has found that most women are completely confused about how much they should eat in pregnancy. In fact, when expectant mums were questioned about their nutritional needs, only a third knew and understood the recommended guidelines.

It's understandable. The headlines, health research and advice from family and friends can be conflicting and confusing. In fact, the National Institute for Clinical Excellence (NICE) suggests that women don't need any extra calories for the first six months of pregnancy and even in the last trimester they only need a paltry two hundred extra calories a day, that's a couple of slices of toast with spread, so it is a long, long way from 'eating for two.'

It's a matter of energy balance. For every 3,500 calories you eat over and above your needs, you could gain a pound of fat. The sad truth is that if you double your intake, you'll end up with a load of excess weight which will be difficult to lose and isn't healthy for you or your baby.

Dr Keith says:

The average woman needs to eat about 2,000 calories daily, depending on her size and level of activity.

- In pregnancy, no extra calories are needed for the first six months.
- In the final trimester, a woman needs 200 more calories a day.
- Every 3,500 calories consumed above your needs could mean a pound of fat gained.

If you were planning on using pregnancy as an excuse to indulge in your favourite forbidden foods, think again. In recent research, more than a quarter of pregnant women admitted they used eating for two as an excuse to eat unhealthy foods but they could be putting their health as well as that of their babies at risk. Professor Janice Rymer, Vice President of Education for the Royal College of Obstetricians and Gynaecologists, said that eating too much while pregnant can harm both mother and child:

Women who are overweight during pregnancy are at an increased risk of having a miscarriage and developing conditions such as gestational diabetes, high blood pressure and pre-eclampsia. They are also more likely to have a premature baby, require a Caesarean section, experience a haemorrhage after birth or develop a clot which can be life-threatening. In addition, overweight women have bigger babies who are themselves more likely to become obese and have significant health problems as a result.

Nourishment for you and your baby

Your baby will need lots of vitamins and minerals to drive their growth and development. Your body becomes more efficient and extracting the goodness out of the food you eat, but it's still important to choose a healthy, balanced and varied diet.

So instead of eating more, you need to eat better. I know that can be tricky. When you're fighting the nausea, heartburn and total exhaustion of early pregnancy, cooking nutritious balanced meals may not be a priority. You may know that salmon and broccoli is better for you and your baby—but when you're dealing with sickness, a packet of biscuits can seem much more appealing.

Try to enjoy food from the five main groups of fruit and veggies, carbohydrates—especially complex and wholegrain carbs like porridge and brown rice—protein from fish, eggs, meat and pulses, dairy such as milk and yoghurt, and healthy fats such as nuts, avocado and oily fish. Limit processed foods and stay away from snacks and drinks that are high in fat and sugar like fizzy drinks, cookies and cakes. Instead, choose healthy snacks such as salad vegetables, hummus, and vegetable soup. (Source: NHS Choices)

What about those extra two hundred calories?

Snack on nutrient-rich foods like:

- Carrot and pita strips dipped in hummus
- Mini egg frittatas with leek, cheese and ham
- Full fat Greek yoghurt with berries and a sprinkling of nuts
- Avocado on wholemeal toast
- Boiled egg and rye soldiers
- Cheese chunks, apple slices and almonds

Or, of course, you could get your extra calories in a Mars Bar and swill down a multivitamin but I think you probably know that's not the best bang for your calorie buck!

> *I'd definitely advise people to try, try, try to be sensible during pregnancy. Once the baby comes it is hard to find time to exercise and eat proper meals. I did try to be a lot more sensible with my second pregnancy and included lots of iron and vitamins in my diet—but towards the end, you get so fed up and eat whatever's around you. I regret that. I've got lots of weight to lose now and I want to be healthy to run after my boys.*
>
> **~ Lindsey, Kilkeel**

> *I don't feel like I ate any more while being pregnant. I ate as normal and tried to eat a bit healthier and drink more water. In my first three months of pregnancy, I found I felt extremely sick until I ate something and then my sickness subsided, I made sure I was eating enough to combat the sickness. I feel I gained the right amount of weight and lost it after giving birth. It was definitely not as quick the second time around, though!*
>
> **~ Sam, Northfields**

The real message is that in pregnancy you need to eat better, not more. With a nutrient-packed diet, you can feel fantastic, maintain your own body's wellbeing and build a healthy baby.

Dr Keith's top five healthy eating tips

Eating in pregnancy is about more than just getting enough energy to keep your body functioning. Your nutritional status can affect your health during pregnancy as well as your baby. A balanced diet with essential supplements can maintain your own wellbeing and help reduce the risk of having a baby with a birth defect.

Start from firm foundations

A scary 40% of British women have an unhealthy diet, so they are already lacking essential vitamins and minerals when they get pregnant. Researcher Professor John Challis, of the University of Toronto, said:

Women need to think about proper diet and food intake before they even know they're pregnant because proper nutrition after pregnancy may not compensate for the lack of it beforehand. Even a modest restriction around the time of conception could have far-reaching consequences.

It's a great idea to think about your nutrition well before you chuck away your contraception. Remember to start taking a 400 microgram folic acid supplement as soon as you start trying to conceive; it's been proven to help protect against neural tube defects like spina bifida.

Boost your blood

Your body has to make extra blood to support your developing baby and this can put a strain on your iron stores. When you consider that heavy periods, dieting and poor nutrition mean that many women are lacking iron when they conceive, it's not surprising anaemia is a common problem.

Beat it by tucking into green leafy vegetables and watercress, red meat and dark meat from poultry, and dried fruits such as apricots. Vitamin C, from citrus fruits, kiwis, tomatoes and fresh juices, will help your body absorb more iron from the vegetables in your diet.

Break the fast

Breakfast goes in and out of fashion. For many years, it was thought to be the most important meal of the day. Then intermittent fasting and 16:8 diet schemes sent it back out of favour. In pregnancy, it's important to start the day well. A good breakfast can boost your energy levels and settle your stomach if nausea is a problem. Think about eating protein, healthy fats, dairy and wholegrains for a nutritional boost. Try scrambled eggs with pumpernickel toast, avocado on rye bread or Greek yoghurt with berries and nuts.

Pack in the fibre providers

Constipation is a common problem, affecting around half of pregnant women. It can leave you cross and crampy and it can also predispose to piles, which aren't on the top of anyone's wish list!

The good news is you can keep your bowels relaxed and regular by looking carefully at the food you eat. Pulses and beans, wholegrains like oats, plenty of fruit and veggies and loads of water will keep your stool soft and your bowels moving.

Stock up on supplements

If I could wave a wand, I'd ensure that every pregnant woman gets the nutrients they need from a healthy balanced diet. But when you're sick, tired and struggling to juggle work and home life, it can be difficult to eat as well as you should.

We also know that the amount of folic acid needed in the early months of pregnancy is nearly four times the usual level. Unless you plan on mainlining Brussel sprouts at a rate of fifteen extra servings a day, it's simply not possible to get everything you need from your food.

Vitamin D is another essential micronutrient that is worryingly lacking in many Northern Europeans. It's found in oily fish and dairy produce and we can even make it ourselves in the presence of sunlight. But gloomy weather, too little time outdoors and poor diets mean that many people are lacking in this vitamin that is so important to enable your baby to develop strong bones and healthy muscles.

It can be sensible to take a pregnancy multivitamin to provide the folic acid and vitamin D you need as well as the reassurance that you're getting the other vitamins and minerals essential for the healthy growth and development of your baby.

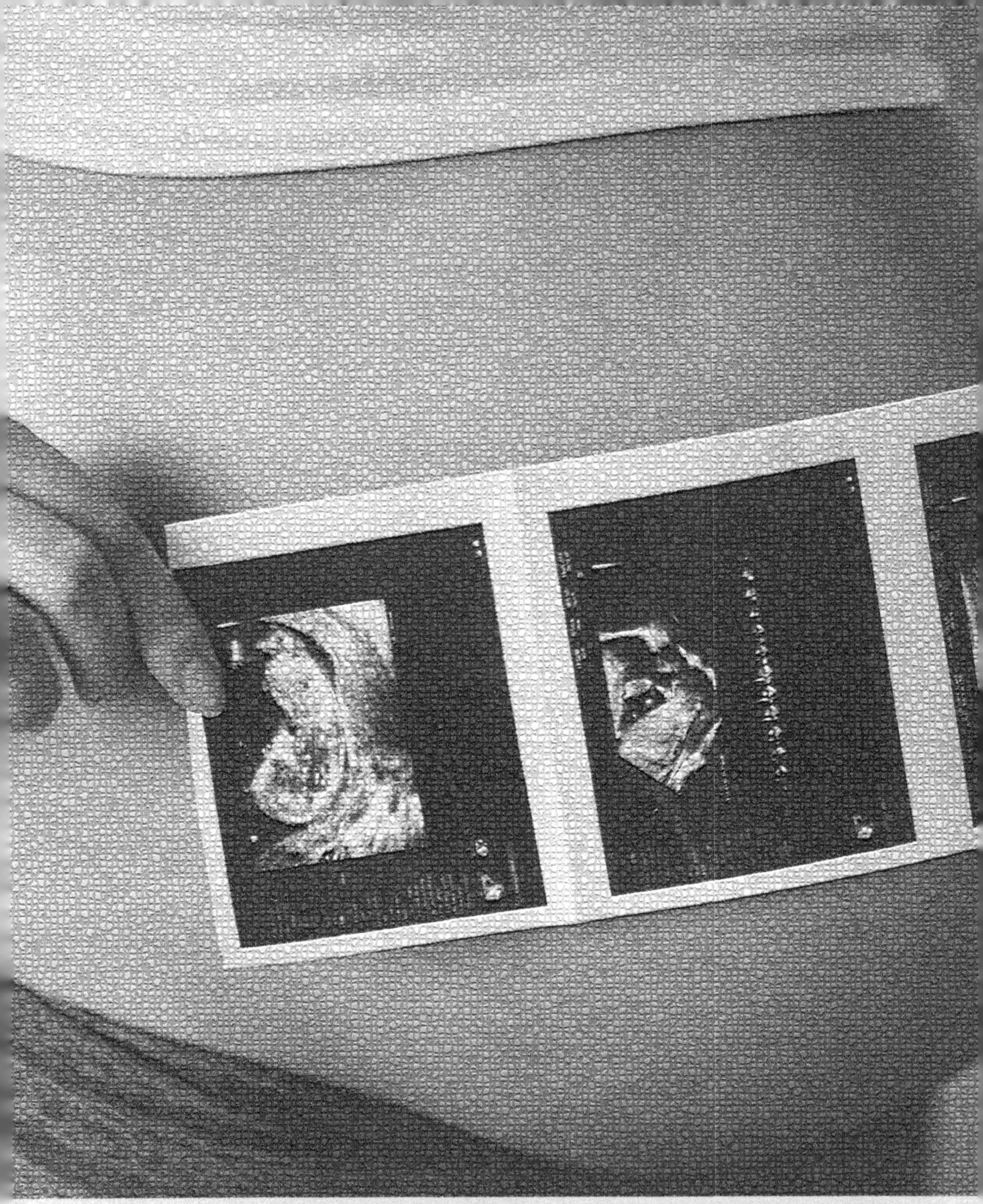

"Most women feel their baby's first movements between 18 and 20 weeks. It's known as the quickening."

23

HOW SOON WILL I FEEL MY BABY'S FIRST MOVEMENTS?

There are few things more magical than feeling the first gentle butterfly flutters of your baby's movements. Suddenly, this is not a bundle of cells; this a living, growing, moving human.

Most women first notice their baby moving between 18 and 20 weeks. They're soft in the early days and it's easy to mistake them for wind. Women who are on their first pregnancy may not spot them until after 20 weeks, while experienced mums can sometimes pick them up as early as 16 weeks.

Rocking and rolling

Depending on the way your baby's moving, the stage of development and your own senses, you may feel a swish, a flutter, a roll or a good hard kick. As your baby grows and develops, you may notice times when they snooze and when they really flex their muscles. The afternoon and evening are often times of peak activity. In between, your baby will nap regularly for between twenty and forty minutes. It's normal not to feel movements during these periods, however they rarely sleep for more than ninety minutes.

The number of movements tend to increase until 32 weeks and then stay stable. An active baby is usually a healthy one, and they should keep on kicking right up to delivery.

Movement matters

Feeling your baby move is their communication with you, providing the comfort and reassurance that they're active and well. There is no normal number of movements that you need to tick off. Instead, try to get to know your baby's personal pattern of movement. If you notice a decrease or a change, it could indicate they may be unwell.

Sometimes you'll be too busy to notice movement, even though they're kicking away merrily. You may also feel fewer flutters if the baby is lying with their back along the front of the uterus. They'll be happily jiggling away inside, but it can be more difficult for you to actually feel the sensations.

Dr Keith says:

Don't worry if your baby is moving like mad. It doesn't mean it is in distress; babies who are in distress stay still.

Placental position

When the placenta develops on the front wall of the womb (anterior placenta) it can sometimes cushion you from feeling your baby's movements. Your little one can be wriggling away frantically but you may not feel it. It can mean there's a delay before you feel the first flutters and you'll notice less movement in the second trimester until their little legs are strong enough to kick on through.

Why is my baby moving less?

Painkillers, sedatives and alcohol can make your baby drowsy and less active.

Sometimes, a baby may move less because they are unwell or in distress. There are also rare conditions that affect the nerves and muscle and make it difficult for your baby to move.

What should I do if I feel decreased movements?

Get help immediately if you're worried about your baby's movements. By acting quickly your medical team can identify if there are any signs of distress, bring on early delivery if your baby is struggling and potentially save their life.

If you're unsure if the movements have really reduced, it's a good idea to lie down on your left side and totally concentrate on your baby for two hours. If you don't feel at least ten separate movements, you should get medical help.

Mum's conundrum

My baby seems to sleep a lot more at the moment and they're definitely not moving around as much, is that normal towards the end of pregnancy or should I be worried?

~ Hannah, Cardiff

Dr Keith says:

The wriggles and kicks of your baby's movements are a tangible sign of the living human being growing inside your womb. Yes, your baby will take time to rest and snooze, and the movements may change in character as they get bigger and space gets a little tight, but your little one really should remain active right up to the birth.

It's great you're aware of their pattern of activity but it's important to seek help if there's a noticeable reduction. If you're unsure, lie down on your left side and focus on counting the kicks, but I recommend getting help sooner rather than later.

Don't wait and sleep on it, speak to your midwife, your doctor or the labour ward straight away. It doesn't matter what time of the day or night it is.

What will happen?

No matter what stage of your pregnancy, your healthcare team will be able to check that all is well with your baby.

Before 24 weeks: If by this stage you still haven't felt movement, you should get in touch with your doctor or your midwife. They'll be able to listen to the baby's heartbeat, arrange an ultrasound scan or consider a referral to a fetal medicine expert like myself to check that your baby is healthy and well.

From 24 weeks to 28 weeks: Contact your doctor or midwife, who will be able to do a full check-up of the baby's heartbeat, the size of your womb, your blood pressure and your urine. If you're measuring a little small, an ultrasound will be organised to assess your baby's growth and development.

> *I had a few scares in pregnancy due to lack of movement. I was told that if ever I was concerned, to drink coke as the sugar should wake the baby up and then obviously if there was still no movement then I should take a trip to the hospital. I don't know if that's right, but it seemed to work.*
>
> **~ Kirsty, Annalong**

After 28 weeks: Call your doctor, your midwife or your maternity unit straight away. You will be asked the details of your baby's movements. You will probably be called in for a full antenatal check-up. They will monitor your baby's heartbeat for at least twenty minutes. This will hopefully confirm their wellbeing and reassure you they are still healthy and kicking.

An ultrasound scan may be arranged if your womb measures smaller than expected or you are at risk of complications because you have high blood pressure, diabetes or have had bleeding in pregnancy.

It's a frightening and stressful time, but I'd like to reassure you, as someone who regularly works in a fetal medicine unit, most women who experience one episode of reduction in their baby's movements have a straightforward pregnancy and go on to deliver wonderful, healthy babies.

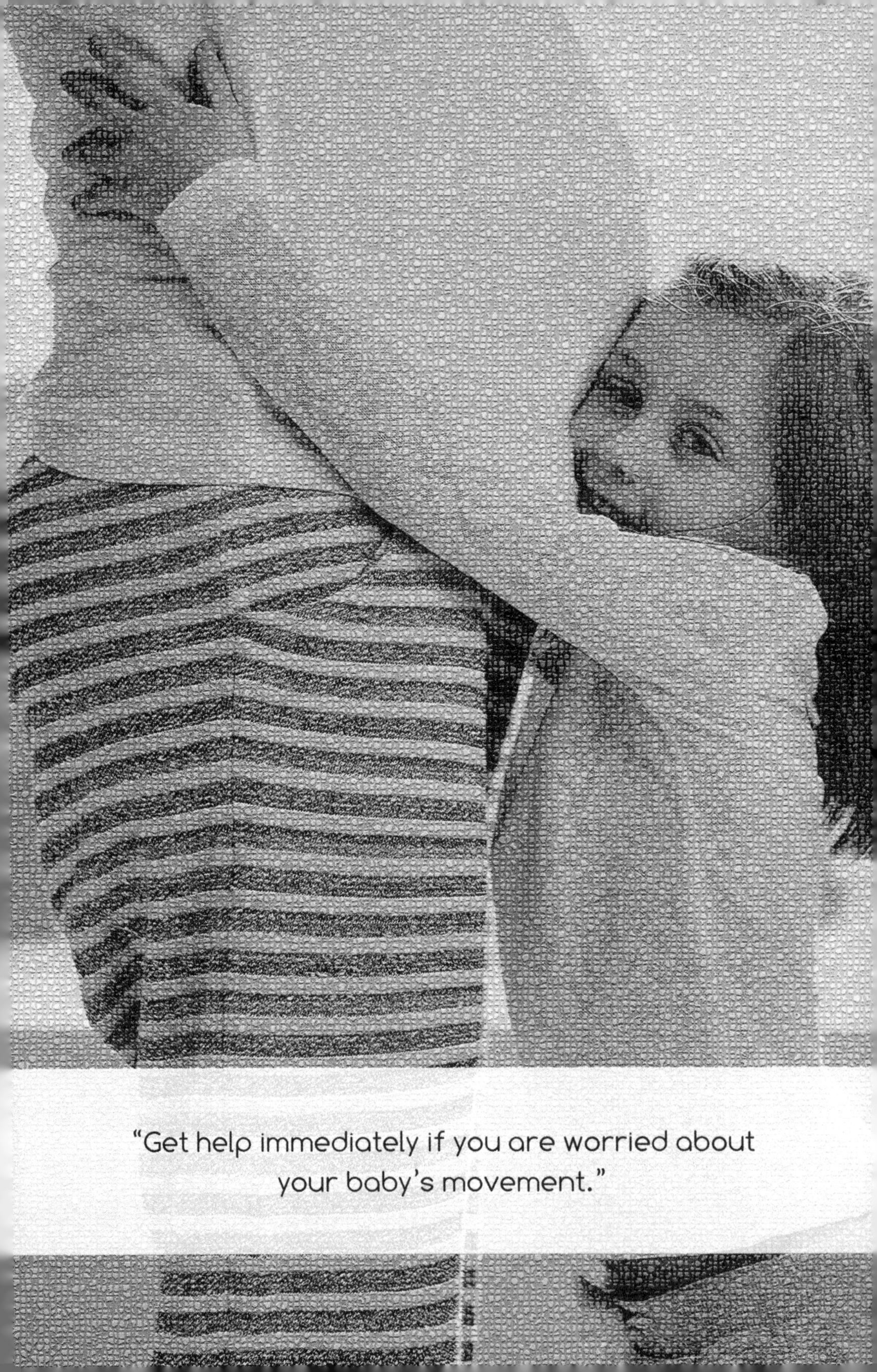

"Get help immediately if you are worried about your baby's movement."

24

HOW DO I KNOW MY BABY WILL BE OK?

Throughout pregnancy, you will be offered a number of routine tests and checks to keep a close eye on your health and the development and wellbeing of the little life growing inside you.

These tests are not compulsory, so you can choose to refuse them if you wish. They are, however incredibly useful to help identify problems and to monitor and treat any complications as promptly as possible. Your doctor should talk through the reasons for any tests, so you can assess the pros and cons and make an informed and intelligent choice.

At each antenatal appointment, you'll have a blood pressure measurement to check for pre-eclampsia, and a urine test to look for blood, protein and glucose. These can be an indication of infection, pre-eclampsia and gestational diabetes. You'll also be offered a number of blood tests to monitor your wellbeing throughout your pregnancy.

Checking your baby's growth

As your baby grows, your bump will expand too. Your doctor or midwife can keep a close eye on their healthy development by measuring the size of your bump. By 20 weeks the womb will have reached your tummy button. That's a convenient 20 centimetres from your pubic bone. It will continue to swell by a centimetre a week, so these measurements can be plotted on a graph to show a safe and steady pattern of growth, or to quickly identify any problems so your baby can have further investigations.

Doppler scans

Whenever we spot growth problems, it's important to keep a close eye on the baby, especially towards the end of pregnancy. A scan may be arranged to repeat the measurements. If there are concerns, a Doppler scan may also be offered. That's a special type of ultrasound that measures blood flow in different parts of the baby, including the umbilical cord, the brain, and the heart.

A scan can give us a much better idea of how well the placenta is functioning. The placenta is the baby's life-support machine. If blood flow is decreased, the baby won't be getting the nutrition they need. That can significantly affect their growth, so we have to consider whether they are still safe within the womb and balance that against the risks of a premature birth. Sometimes the baby may be better off if they are delivered early.

Abdominal examination

The experienced hands of your pregnancy doctor or midwife can provide an enormous amount of information about the baby growing in your womb. They can identify movements, check position and see whether their head has started to move down into the pelvis ready for birth. They will also listen to the magical thump of your baby's heartbeat using a stethoscope or hand-held Doppler device.

In addition to these routine checks and measures you will also be offered a number of other screening tests and scans, or if you are thought to be at risk due to your age, your family or your medical history, diagnostic tests to identify certain genetic or chromosomal conditions may be suggested.

Your pregnancy ultrasound scans

The monochrome ultrasound images of your baby's dating scan usually offer the first picture of your beautiful baby. I say beautiful, but try to remember that ultrasound uses sound waves to develop an image of your baby. The waves bounce back from solid objects like bone and pass through liquids, so the scan sees all the way through your baby's skin to show the internal organs and structures. Believe me, all babies look a little like extras from Lord of the Rings!

Scans provide fantastic information; I can check the chambers of the heart, look for cleft lip and palate and examine the fold of fluid behind the neck. But it's not useful if you'd like to see a picture of your baby looking like... well, a baby.

Sometimes silence is scary during a scan, but it is mostly concentration on their part. One doctor thought my baby was measuring quite small and made me have more appointments than usual, but I asked plenty of questions to get reassurance that all was OK. That would be my piece of advice—if you feel unsettled, or have a question, ask it. Don't feel silly or whatever—your baby is the most important thing and it's important you understand what is happening to it and to you!

~ Lindsey, Kilkeel

In the UK, pregnant women are offered at least two ultrasound scans during their pregnancy:

- **The dating scan**: This ultrasound is carried out between 8 and 14 weeks. Your doctor or sonographer will check your pregnancy is progressing well, take a look to see if more than one baby is nestling in your womb and carefully measure the baby so the estimated date of delivery can be calculated.

  At this stage, a fold of fluid at the back of the neck called the nuchal fold may also be measured as part of the combined screening test for Down's syndrome.

- **The anomaly scan**: This is a more detailed scan offered to every pregnant woman between 18 and 21 weeks. The sonographer will check that your baby has continued to grow at a healthy rate and will also check for any structural abnormalities. They will examine the chambers of the heart, the organs, the spine and the limbs and they'll also look at the face to check for cleft lip and palate. The scan will also show the position your baby is lying in and the location of the placenta.

At my second scan at twenty weeks they picked up potential placenta praevia. It was frightening because I didn't know what this was, and the sonographer didn't give me much information. I was booked in for an extra scan for this at thirty-two weeks and then thirty-six weeks, when the placenta finally moved enough to have a natural birth.

~ Sam, Northfield

Boy or girl?

To know, or not to know, that is the question. Your doctor or scanner will check your baby's genitals but actually discovering the sex of your baby isn't part of the screening programme. However, different hospitals have different policies. If you'd like to know, ask the sonographer at the beginning of the scan.

But, be warned, even if they're happy to look it's not always possible to tell. Your baby may be demurely crossing their legs; they may be in an awkward position or it may be tricky to tell. Take my advice and don't splash out too much on pink or blue baby-grows unless they're really confident.

Can I have someone with me?

Having a scan can be an exciting but also a frightening time. You may be able to see your little one waving at you or sucking their thumb. Sadly, some people discover that there are problems with the baby, so it's a good idea to have a friend, partner or family member with you when you attend to provide support. There's not usually any childcare available, so it's important to arrange for someone to babysit any other children.

When will I get the results?

The results are immediate and the sonographer is usually able to tell you everything on the day. However, if they are struggling to see some details clearly or are concerned there may be a problem, they may ask for a second opinion. Sometimes you will be offered further tests, scans or a referral to a specialist fetal medicine consultant, like myself, to find out more.

Say cheese!

At most hospitals, you can get a printed picture of your scan, although there is often a small charge. Check with your unit for their policy and you'll have the first picture for your new family album.

Can I say no?

Ultrasound scans are considered safe for both mum and baby and can provide useful information. However, you don't have to have a scan, and if you refuse your choice will be respected.

If you are uncertain about scans because you know you will proceed with the pregnancy, no matter what anomalies and problems are shown, it is worth chatting through your concerns with your midwife or doctor. Scans are about much more than looking for abnormalities. They can also provide accurate information about the position of the placenta, whether you're having twins and your baby's growth. Put simply, they will help increase the chance of you delivering your baby safely.

Testing for chromosomal abnormalities

Chromosomes are long, thread-like structures made up of DNA and proteins. They store the genetic information that controls everything from the colour of our eyes, to our sex and our tendency to develop disease. Sometimes there can be problems with the chromosomes, leading to babies being born with syndromes that can affect their appearance, health and intelligence.

Screening can provide you with early information about your specific risk of having a baby with damaged or extra chromosomes. Knowledge gleaned from scans and blood-tests can be used to determine your risk of carrying a baby with the more common of these conditions, these include:

- **Down's syndrome**, where there is an extra copy of chromosome 21, known as trisomy 21
- **Edward's syndrome**, where there is an extra copy of chromosome 18, or trisomy 21
- **Patau's syndrome**, which is trisomy 13.

Screening

In the UK, screening tests are offered at around 12 weeks. However, if you book a little later, there are alternative options.

The combined test

The combined test is done when you are between 11 and 14 weeks pregnant. You will have a blood test to check for specific proteins in your blood, and an ultrasound scan, in which a specific fold of fluid that's found behind your baby's neck is measured. The blood test results, together with the information from the **nuchal translucency** scan are combined with your risk factors and your age to calculate your statistical risk of having a baby with a chromosomal condition.

The quadruple test

The quadruple test can be performed later than the combined test, so it can be used if you have booked late. It is ideally done between 16 and 19 weeks, although it can sometimes be carried out as late as 22 weeks if necessary. The clue is in the name; it's a blood test that tests for four different proteins. The results are fed into a computer programme, together with your age and other risk-factors, to work out the likelihood of your baby being affected by a chromosomal abnormality.

Non-invasive prenatal testing

NIPT is a new, simple blood test that can detect fetal cells in the maternal circulation. These cells can be tested to find out the baby's sex and to check for chromosomal abnormalities like Down's syndrome. Although it is a screening test, it can accurately identify Down's in 99.9% of cases.

A matter of choice

Remember, you don't have to have these tests. And if you do get a positive result, it doesn't mean that there will be any pressure to have further investigations or to terminate. Instead, it can be an opportunity to think, talk to your partner and make a considered choice that's right for your family.

25

ARE SCREENING TESTS ALWAYS RIGHT?

The barrage of tests in pregnancy can sometimes seem overwhelming. The what, when and whys can be confusing and it can be difficult to know how helpful and accurate they are.

Screening tests will not tell you whether your baby has a chromosomal condition or not. They can only tell you the statistical chance of your baby being affected. Based on the results of tests, together with your age and other risk factors, the risk that your baby has a specific condition, such as Down's syndrome will be calculated. The results of any screening test won't tell you for sure that your baby is affected. Instead, they'll give you a statistical figure of their risk.

What is risk?

The idea of risk can be tricky to understand. It really refers to the chance of something happening. So you'll be given a risk of, say, 1 in 100 or 1%. This means that for every hundred women who had this test result, only one would have a baby affected by Down's. The other 99 babies would be unaffected.

Your doctor should help you understand the implications of the result and help you make the decision whether to have further more definitive tests. Sometimes, your healthcare professional may refer to your screening test as being positive. This does not mean your baby is definitely affected; it simply means that their risk is higher than the cut off when a diagnostic test is recommended, often this is set at the level at which the danger to the baby of having the diagnostic test is higher than the risk of the condition.

No screening test is totally accurate and tests inevitably miss some babies that are affected and wrongly identify some that aren't. For example, research suggests that the combined screening test is able to pick up nine in ten babies with Down's syndrome but it also gives false positives in one in twenty cases.

Examples of screening tests include the tests discussed in the previous section:

- **The combined test for Down's syndrome**
- **The quadruple test**
- **NIPT**

Diagnostic tests

Unlike screening tests, diagnostic tests look at direct genetic material from your baby and so are able to accurately diagnose chromosomal abnormalities. They are usually carried out on women who are at increased risk of having a baby with a genetic issue. This could be because a screening test indicated an increased risk, because you're over the age of thirty-five or because a genetic condition is thought to run in the family.

The diagnostic tests include amniocentesis and chorionic villus sampling. Unfortunately, these are invasive investigations, which carries risks to your baby:

- **Chorionic villus sampling (CVS)** is a diagnostic test to identify chromosomal problems affecting the baby. The test is done by putting a small tube into your uterus through the vagina or putting a needle into the uterus, through the skin on the lower abdomen, to take cells from the tiny fi nger-like projections on the placenta called the chorionic villi. The sample is sent to a lab for genetic analysis, to produce a *karyotype*, which is a picture of your baby's chromosomes, so your doctor can see for sure if there are any problems.

  The results are much more accurate than screening tests, detecting abnormalities with 98 per cent accuracy. However, as it is more invasive it carries more risks, including the risk of miscarriage

- **Amniocentesis** is a special kind of diagnostic test that looks at genetic material from the fluid surrounding your baby, so any chromosomal abnormalities can be identified. Amniocentesis is most often done during the second trimester, after 15 weeks. It is usually carried out on women who have been identified as being at risk of having a baby with a genetic condition like Down's syndrome.

  Using ultrasound to guide the procedure, an expert will insert a long, thin needle through the skin of your abdomen. It will go through the wall of the womb and into the sac around your baby. A small amount of the amniotic fluid will be withdrawn for analysis.

A karyotype of your baby's chromosomal make-up will be made to definitively identify any problems. Sadly, between one and two in two hundred women will have a miscarriage following the procedure, often because of the introduction of infection at the time of the test.

Non-invasive prenatal screening test (NIPT)

NIPT is a new type of super-sensitive screening test. The test involves an ultrasound scan to check your dates and a blood test to look at the small amount of your baby's DNA that can be found in your blood. It can be carried out from 10 weeks until the end of pregnancy. It can check the risk of Down's syndrome as well as other conditions like Edward's and Patau's.

The term non-invasive refers to the simplicity and safety of the test, as compared to invasive tests like amniocentesis and CVS, which carry a risk of miscarriage. Although it is not a diagnostic test, it has been shown to have a pick-up rate of 99.9% for Down's syndrome.

Scans are not always right

I measured several weeks ahead for most of my pregnancy and as a result was tested for diabetes, which fortunately I didn't have. I had several growth scans towards the end of my pregnancy telling me that my baby was massive. In the end, Sophia was eight pounds five ounces when she was born, so just a normal size.

~ Kirsty, Annalong

The right choice for you

Only you and your partner can decide whether you want to have screening or diagnostic tests. I work every day scanning pregnant women and checking for abnormalities in babies, so I know how valuable these tests can be. Yet, when my wife Sharon was pregnant we decided not to have diagnostic chromosomal tests. We knew that whatever happened with our baby, whatever problems she faced, we wanted to proceed with the pregnancy and were more comfortable watching and waiting. There is no right way; just the best one for you.

THE THIRD TRIMESTER

"The end of your pregnancy is in sight.
It won't be long until your baby arrives."

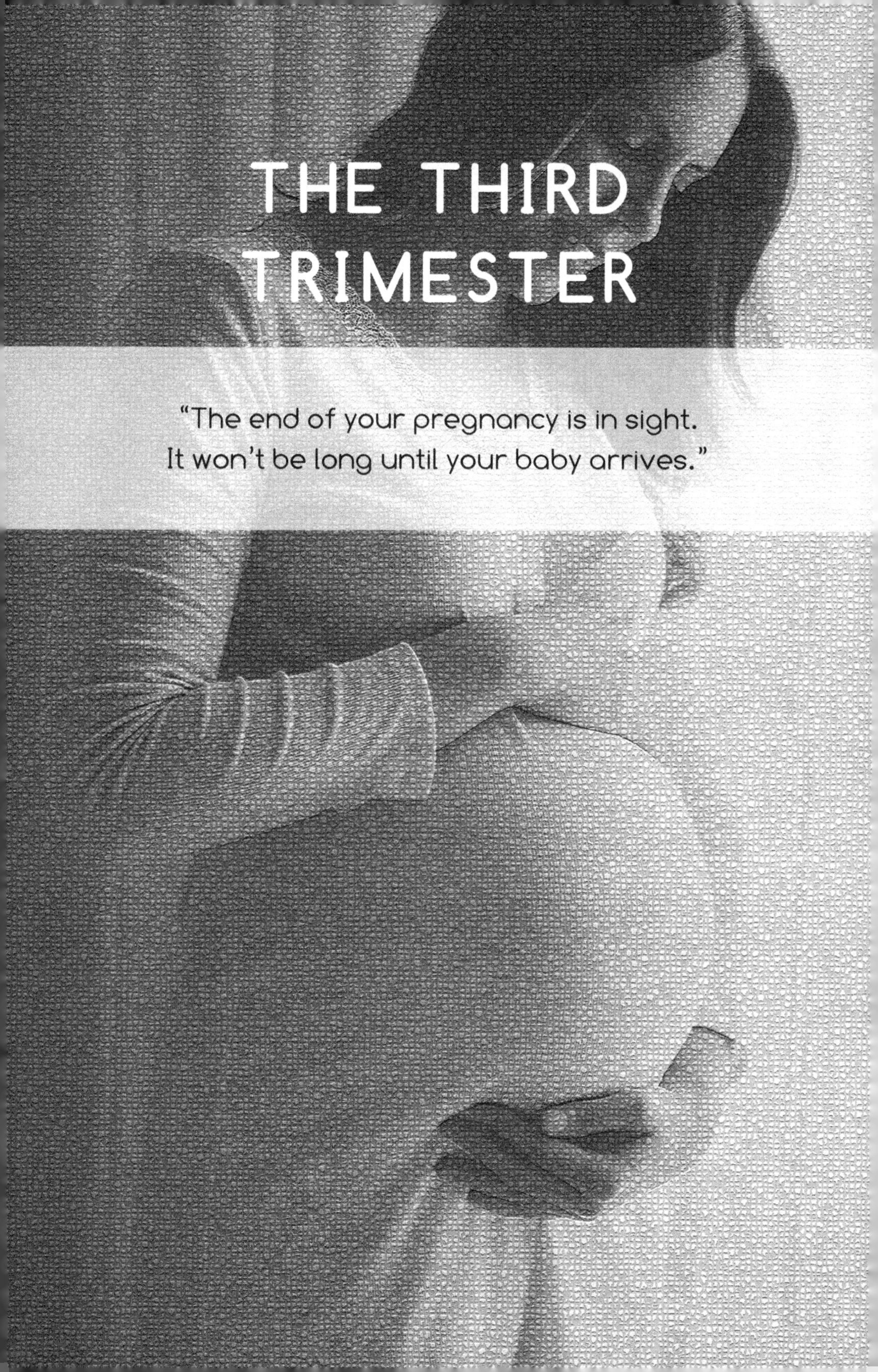

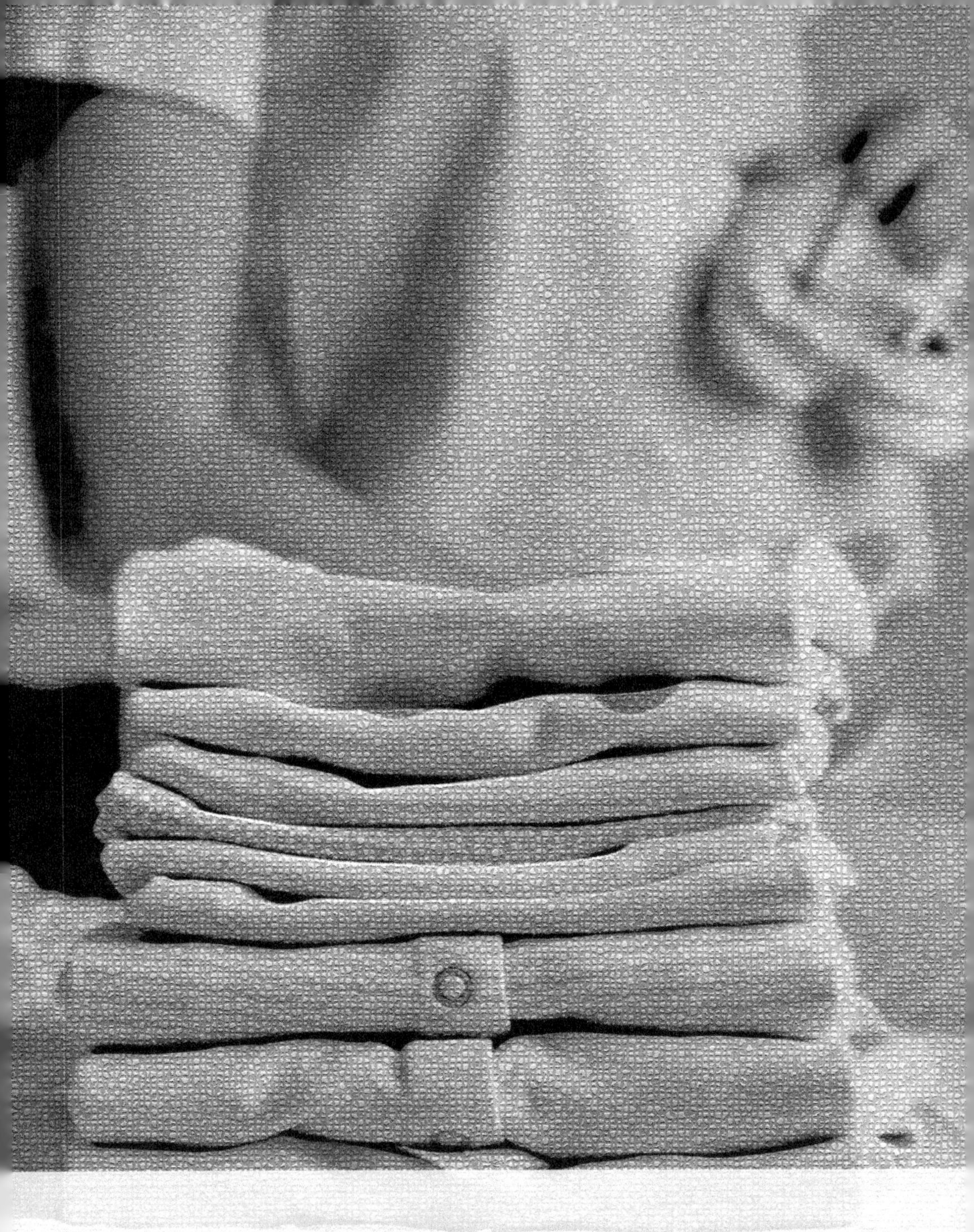

"A little puffiness is part and parcel of pregnancy—but get medical help if it is painful or comes on suddenly."

26

WHY ARE MY LEGS SO SWOLLEN?

Ankle swelling is common in the later stages of pregnancy. In fact, as many as three quarters of women find they get a little puffy. It's usually worse when it's warm or if you've been standing for long periods.

The medical term for swelling is oedema. It's down to your body retaining fluid because of your increased blood flow and your womb pressing down on the vein that returns blood to your heart. The fluid leaks from the bloodstream into the tissues and gravity makes it collect in your hands and feet.

It's a totally normal condition, but it can be annoying when your rings and shoes no longer fit, and your lovely legs look like more like tree trunks. However, there are a few things you can try to ease oedema:

- Sip water regularly to stay well hydrated, keep your system flushed and prevent water retention
- Put your feet up and relax for a while; it'll help the fluid drain away

- Try not to stand still for long periods
- Don't cross your legs, it can make swelling worse
- Exercise the area by rotating your ankles or wrists, to help any extra fluid drain away

Towards the end of both my pregnancies I got terrible cankles. The only shoes I could wear were Uggs and Crocs! I used it as an excellent excuse to put my feet up in front of the TV and get my partner to run around after me!

~ Louise, York

When swelling could be serious

A little puffiness is part and parcel of pregnancy, but sometimes swelling can be more than an irritation. It's essential to get medical help if it's extensive or if it comes on suddenly. You may be suffering from a condition called pre-eclampsia.

Pre-eclampsia

Pre-eclampsia is a serious pregnancy complication in which your blood pressure becomes dangerously high. It combines hypertension, protein in your urine and sometimes sudden and alarming swelling. The condition affects as many as one in ten pregnancies and can have severe consequences for you and your baby if it's not treated and controlled promptly.

The good news is that your midwife and doctor will be well aware of the dangers of pre-eclampsia and will monitor you throughout pregnancy. However, it can sometimes come on suddenly, in between clinic appointments, so it's important to be aware of the signs and symptoms. If you're alert and informed, you can get medical help urgently if you become unwell and protect your health as well as that of your baby.

Signs and symptoms

Very often women with pre-eclampsia can feel perfectly well at first, even though their blood pressure may be sky high. However, pregnancy hypertension may be associated with:

- **Swelling**: this can come on suddenly and affect your ankles, legs, face and hands. Sometimes you may feel as if your whole body has puffed up.
- **Headache**: this can be severe and relentless and doesn't go away with paracetamol.
- **Visual disturbances**: such as blurring or flashing.
- **Abdominal pain**: this can be strong and sharp below the ribs.

It's important to contact your healthcare team urgently if you notice any of these symptoms. Remember, things can change rapidly in pregnancy. It's worth getting checked, even if your blood-pressure has been recently measured.

Who is at risk?

Anyone can get pre-eclampsia, so don't be complacent and ignore the signs. However, some people are more at risk. This includes women:

- In their first pregnancy and those who are under eighteen or over forty
- With a previous history of pre-eclampsia or a family history of the condition
- Having twins or more
- With a history of hypertension
- With kidney disease, or autoimmune conditions like rheumatoid arthritis and lupus
- Who are obese with a BMI over 30
- With polycystic ovarian syndrome
- Who have become pregnant through IVF

Checks and measures

If you are at high risk of developing pre-eclampsia, your doctor will keep a close eye on you and your baby. Every pregnant woman will be checked throughout pregnancy for the signs of pre-eclampsia. That's why monitoring your blood pressure is such an important part of antenatal care—the first sign of pre-eclampsia is commonly a rise in blood pressure.

As well as regular blood pressure checks, your urine will be checked at each appointment. If you are developing pre-eclampsia, your kidneys may start to leak protein, which may be identified on the dipstick test.

The dangers of high blood pressure in pregnancy

High blood pressure can cause growth problems in your baby and affect their development. If left untreated, pre-eclampsia can develop into a dangerous condition called eclampsia, which may put both you and your baby at risk. It is characterised by uncontrolled blood pressure, fits, brain haemorrhage and retinal detachments in the mother. Sadly, in rare cases, it can lead to the death of the mum or the baby. That's why it's so important to attend your antenatal check-ups and see your doctor if you develop any symptoms. If pre-eclampsia is identified early, the condition can often be monitored and managed to maintain the safety of both mother and child.

Management and medication

Management of your pre-eclampsia will depend on your blood-pressure, your wellbeing, the health of your baby and your stage of pregnancy.

Treatment of pre-eclampsia may include admission, bed rest and medication to reduce your blood pressure. Depending on your health, and your baby's stage of development, you may be prescribed small doses of aspirin to thin your blood. You will need close heart and fetal monitoring, and sometimes a medication called magnesium sulphate may slow the onset of pre-eclampsia, although this works only in the short-term.

The only real cure is delivery of your baby, so if your pre-eclampsia is severe and uncontrolled, you may need to be induced or have an emergency Caesarean to deliver your baby and control the condition. Your baby may need medication to speed up the development of their lungs and reduce the risks of a premature delivery.

If pre-eclampsia comes on when you're already in labour, pain relief from an epidural can help drop the blood pressure a little. The good news is that it is highly likely that your body and your blood pressure will return to normal after the birth.

Most of the women I care for who suffer from pre-eclampsia during their pregnancy have no lasting repercussions, though many will require medication for six weeks or so.

HELLP Syndrome

The name of HELLP Syndrome makes it sound serious, and it is a severe but thankfully uncommon condition affecting the liver and the blood's ability to clot effectively. HELLP syndrome is one of the most severe and dangerous forms of pre-eclampsia, affecting somewhere between one in twenty and one in eight women with pregnancy-induced hypertension.

It usually affects pregnant women immediately after their baby is delivered. But it can appear any time after twenty weeks, and rarely even before that. As well as the classic symptoms of pre-eclampsia (like headache and swelling), a woman may notice severe pain below the ribs on the right. There may also be jaundice and bruising or bleeding, but usually someone would be very unwell by this stage.

HELLP

HELLP is an acronym, with the each of the letters in the name standing for a feature of the syndrome.

Haemolysis: This is a condition in which the red blood cells are broken down.

ELevated liver enzymes: In HELLP the liver enzymes in the blood rise, signalling liver damage.

Low Platelet count: The platelets are the little disc-like particles in the blood that help it to clot, they drop in HELLP potentially leading to haemorrhage.

When you're pregnant, if you feel unwell or have any unexplained or worrying symptoms, it's vital to ask for assessment and advice. Your midwife or doctor will be happy to support and guide you.

The good news is that with the right treatment, women with HELLP can make a full recovery. However, if it comes on before labour, it is essential to deliver the baby as soon as possible.

27

IS IT SAFE TO DYE MY HAIR IN PREGNANCY?

Believe it or not, this is the pregnancy question that I'm asked most often. Lots of expectant mums tell me that the body and skin changes of pregnancy can leave them feeling lumpy and lacking in confidence. If you're used to copper lowlights or a peroxide crop, the idea of having to go back to bland brown or boring mouse can be depressing and demoralising.

The good news is that you're free to tend to your tresses. The chemicals in permanent and semi-permanent hair dyes are not highly toxic. Most of the research evidence (I'll be honest, there isn't loads) shows it's safe to colour your hair while pregnant.

Your crowning glory

Most women notice that their hair is thick, glossy and fabulous in pregnancy. This is because your normal hair shedding cycle has slowed down. Usually, the majority of the hairs on your head are growing while somewhere between five and fifteen per cent are resting. In the normal cycle, the hair that has been resting naturally falls out to be replaced by new fresh growth. That's what's happening when you see hairs on your brush, on the pillow or blocking up the plughole. Most women lose an average of around a hundred hairs a day.

During pregnancy, that process changes. The hormones act to lengthen the growing phase, so less hair is lost. That means that your hair will be thicker. You may also notice that it changes texture and becomes shinier—sometimes curly girls may go straight or vice versa.

Pregnancy can be a great time to experiment and make the most of your locks. However, it's sensible to take a few precautions:

- **Do a strand test**: Your hair may respond differently to bleach or colour, so check how a strand reacts to avoid the Worzel Gummidge look!
- **Do a patch test**: The hormones rampaging around your body can change your response to chemicals and make you more sensitive. So even if it's a colour you've used for years, test first if you don't want a nasty surprise.
- **Get a helping hand**: Ask a hairdresser or a friend to apply the colour so it's quicker, easier and you get less chemical exposure. If that's not possible, wear gloves.
- **Breathe easy**: Put the colour on in a well-ventilated room, so open the window and let the air flood in.
- **Follow the instructions** and don't leave it in for too long before rinsing carefully and thoroughly.

I was afraid to use hair dye, so I didn't colour my hair through most of my pregnancy. Towards the end, the hairdressers put on a safer hair dye and made sure it didn't touch my roots. But I did speak to my midwife after and she said it was perfectly fine to dye my hair.

~ Sam, Northfields

> *I had my hair highlighted twice whilst pregnant. My hairdresser advised because it was highlights and the dye wasn't touching my scalp, then it was totally safe.*
>
> **~ Kirsty, Annalong**

Enjoy your thick mane while it lasts. After the birth, the normal shedding cycle resumes, with a vengeance! More hair will go into the resting phase and then shed, you may notice more hairs falling out meaning blocked plugholes and thinner tresses. Make the most of it now and toss your head—you're worth it!

The things you don't have to give up in pregnancy

Sometimes pregnancy can seem to involve a long list of things that you have to quit. Alcohol, cigarettes, blue cheese and pâté are on the banned list. But that doesn't mean you're facing nine months of misery and self-denial. As well as colouring your hair, there are lots of other little indulgences you can enjoy while building your baby.

Chocolate

In the list of foods to avoid in pregnancy, chocolate is a significant and splendid exception. Yes, it's calorific, but a little of what you fancy really can do you good. Did you know that chocolate has been thought to possess healing powers since ancient times? It has been used to treat all manner of health complaints as well as increasing strength and boosting sexual potency. It also appears that eating chocolate regularly may actually improve the brain's function. Indulge in a little of the dark stuff, but make sure you're not overindulging.

Baths

There's nothing like a deep, warm relaxing bath. It'll take the weight off your bump, ease your muscles and soothe your spirit. Why not try adding a little lavender essential oil or some Epsom Salts to aid relaxation and help you drop off to sleep?

Sex

All the hormones rampaging around the body can make lots of women feel frisky during pregnancy. The good news is that you're free to indulge your desires. It's usually perfectly safe to continue enjoying sex. Check out the next section for more information on pleasure, positions and more.

Massages

A massage can be a wonderful way to ease your aching muscles and knead out the knots. Use a little essential oil and it can either soothe you and send you to sleep or give a boost to your energy and your mood. Choose a therapist with experience in massaging pregnant women, and ask them for a few tips so your partner can repeat the experience at home.

Manicures

Not everyone likes primped and painted fingernails, but if you do, pregnancy could be the perfect time to indulge yourself. Your nails will grow more quickly in pregnancy, and many women find they can be a little harder and less prone to bending, flaking and splitting. Like the changes in your hair, the improvement is temporary. But if you eat well, wear rubber gloves when washing up and moisturise your nailbeds, your fingernails should still be looking great six months after the birth—if you haven't chewed them off with the stress of sleepless nights, that is!

Your morning cuppa

The good news is that you don't have to totally kick the caffeine habit in pregnancy—but you should definitely try to cut down your consumption. It's safe to enjoy up to 200mg of caffeine a day. That's a couple of mugs of instant coffee or around four cups of tea, cheers!

28

DO OLD-WIVES' TALES FOR PREDICTING THE BABY'S SEX WORK?

Girl or boy? Boy or girl? It's the first question everyone asks after their baby has been delivered. Many couples now like to find out their baby's sex at the ultrasound scan, but that doesn't stop everyone from playing guessing games throughout the pregnancy.

When it comes to gender predictions, everyone's an expert. From the shape of your bump, to your choices in the canteen at lunch-time, there are loads of weird and wacky ways of guessing whether your little one's chromosomes are XX or XY. Here are some I've heard of. Why don't you try them and let me know what worked and what didn't?

Bump inspection

Is your bump up front and proud, or wider and more spread out? This is one of the favourite methods, with boys being carried high and forwards and girls being slung a little longer and lower.

Take it from me, I've seen bumps of all shapes and sizes. The way you carry your baby is to do with your muscles, your body and the shape of your pelvis. That little chromosomal difference has nothing to do with it.

> *With both my children people's obsessions with old wives' tales led me to believe I was having girls. Due to the way I carried my second baby, people were convinced I was carrying a girl—in fact, the baby was breech. One friend even swung my engagement ring around my bump on a strand of my hair!*
>
> **~ Amanda, Chichester**

Sugar and spice and all things nice

There's an old wives' tale that says women crave sweet things when they're carrying a girl and salty or savoury stuff when there's a little boy incubating inside.

The key clue

If someone puts a key in front of you, do you reach for the wide end or the pointy one? If you grab the narrow bit, you'll have a girl, the other part and it'll be a boy. Or maybe you grabbed the nearest and easiest to access part, who knows? You've got a fifty-fifty chance of it being right in the end!

Ring, ring

This is an old wives' tale that's fun to try. Slip off your wedding ring and attach it to a long piece of string. Now, let it dangle freely over your bump. If it swings in a circular fashion, start flicking through boy's names. If instead it goes back and for like a pendulum, you should start looking in the girl's section of your name guide.

She makes me sick!

Girls make mums sick. No, really. Well, that's the theory anyway. If morning sickness was a problem in your early pregnancy, you're meant to be more likely to be carrying a girl. If you sailed through, a boy it is. With eight in ten pregnant women suffering from morning sickness, I'm not sure the statistics really back this one up!

Spot the difference

It's also often said that if you're carrying a girl you may be more likely to get spots, pimples and acne. With a boy, your skin will be peachy and perfect. Are you getting the impression from these old wives' tales that when it comes to pregnancy, little girls bring the bad stuff?

Some women do suffer with their skin in pregnancy—but it's more to do with the progesterone pumping through their body than any impact from the tiny bean inside.

Trying for a boy or a girl

The mythology about your baby's gender starts before conception. For thousands of years, parents have tried various tricks and techniques, to try to cheat the odds and make it more likely that they deliver a little boy or a girl. A host of folklore and falsehoods have evolved about the ways and means of affecting that essential chromosomal configuration. But is there any truth behind these traditional tales?

Food

According to old wives' or husbands' tales, your diet at the time of conception can have an impact much lower down in your body. If you want a girl you should indulge in sugar and spice and all things nice, whereas red meat and salty savouries will encourage a little boy. I know we are what we eat, but that really is stretching things a little!

Getting satisfaction

If you want a little boy, make sure your partner pays you plenty of attention in the bedroom! If you reach orgasm, you'll release fluid with an alkaline pH that is thought to favour the male-sperm. It should be more enjoyable too!

Sex for sex

The rumour has been handed down through generations that the way you have sex won't just affect your enjoyment, it can also have an impact on the sex of your baby. Apparently, female sperm cells are slower but longer lasting while the boy sperm are quick but short-lived.

If you want a girl, you should choose a position with shallower penetration, to give the X sperm a better chance of hitting the jackpot. The missionary position, spooning or the lotus flower are perfect. If you want a boy, those Y sperm need to be fired close to the target, so reverse cowgirl or woman on top will help the boy sperm win the race.

Shettles Method

A scientist called Landrum B Shettles developed a system based on a similar premise. It centres on the fact that male sperm are quicker moving but not as long-living as female sperm, but it's about when you have sex, not how. If you want to conceive a boy, you should have sex as near to the time of ovulation as possible. If you want a little girl, you should have sex a few days (2-4) before ovulation. By the time the egg is released, only the X sperm are left, ready to create an XX baby. Shettles claims to have had great results with this technique, saying it works for girls three-quarters of the time and is an extraordinary eighty per cent effective when trying to conceive boys.

Whelan Method

If you're scrabbling for your calendar, your thermometer and some ovulation sticks, hang on. There's another theory devised by a scientist called Elizabeth Whelan. It claims that the hormonal changes early in the menstrual cycle encourage male sperm. So to conceive a boy you need to have sex well before ovulation, around 4-6 days and to have a girl it should be 2-3 days before ovulation. Confused? You're not alone!

The truth is that it is still a matter of chance. Looking at the evidence, it does seem that the Y carrying sperm do have the edge over the X carrying female ones both at the start of the fertile window and at the end. So think about that while you're timing intercourse, but don't paint the nursery blue or pink yet (or do, and rebel against outdated gender stereotyping.)

It's in the stars

The stars, moon and planets have been thought to be imbued with magical powers. If you flick to the horoscopes first in a magazine, you may like to try to harness the powers of astrology when you're trying to conceive.

If you want a girl, make love when the moon is full, or in the afternoon, or on the even days of the month. If you want a boy, do it when there's a quarter moon in the sky, or at night, or on odd days of the month.

Night, day, odd, even. It's like throwing a dice!

The appliance of science

In reality, there's no evidence that anything you try during traditional intercourse can influence which tiny sperm reaches the egg first and fertilises it. It really is a matter of random chance... and a wonderful surprise whether it's a little boy or a little girl.

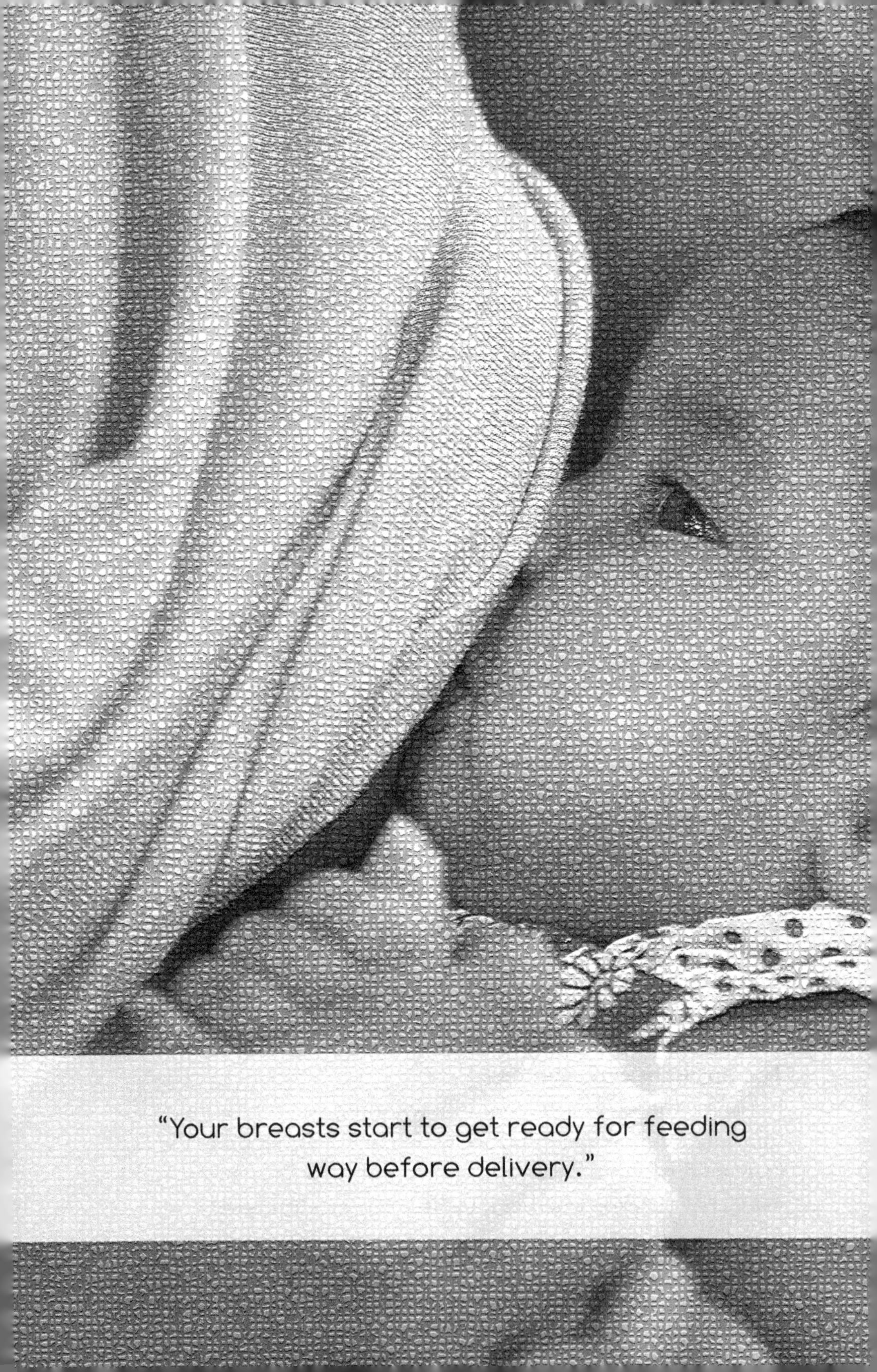

"Your breasts start to get ready for feeding way before delivery."

29

HOW WILL PREGNANCY CHANGE MY BREASTS?

Your breasts have the vital task of providing nourishment for your new baby. They take their job seriously and start adapting even before you've skipped a period. The changes will alter your breasts for life, but with a little care you can keep them comfortable and supported.

Early changes

Pregnancy hormones start to stimulate changes in the breasts early in pregnancy. As soon as a week after conception the blood supply to your breasts is boosted, making your nipples feel tingly and prickly. It could be the first signal that a baby is on the way.

Size matters

By around six weeks you may find your breasts get more tender and sore. As pregnancy progresses you'll notice a definite boost to your cleavage, but your breasts may also feel heavy, swollen and uncomfortable. Many women go up by one or two cup sizes, especially during their first pregnancy.

In vein

The blood supply to your breasts increases and the milk ducts and milk-producing cells develop, so the veins will become more prominent and may be visible as blue or purple lines criss-crossing the surface of your breasts.

Skin stress

Your breasts may feel itchy as your skin stretches, and the hormonal changes together with the rapid increase in size can mean that stretch marks develop. If you're worried about these, have a look at the next section for tips on managing them.

Little leaks

You probably expected a little milk leakage once the baby is born—but your breasts start to get ready for feeding way before the delivery. Many women start to leak colostrum (the first milk) from as early as sixteen weeks. If you're not prepared, it can leave you with two attractive damp patches on your top. The good news is that there are specially designed pads to soak up leaks, so pop some in your bra to avoid the wet t-shirt look.

Nipple news

The changing hormones in your body stimulate a number of alterations in your nipples. You'll notice that they become more pigmented and darker. They may also appear puffy and swollen. It's part of their preparation for the challenges of breastfeeding. Lots of women find them super-sensitive; they can tingle and feel sore in the cold, so keep them warm.

Bumps on bumps

You will have had little bumps on your areolas (the areas around the nipples) before pregnancy. These are glands called Montgomery's tubercles, which release oil to keep your nipples soft, healthy and moisturised. During pregnancy, these may become bigger and more noticeable in preparation for breastfeeding.

My breasts grew massively in pregnancy and the nipples were so big they stuck through my clothes. I used the breast pads to disguise them a little!

~ Jane, Leeds

My breasts increased in size, quite a lot, but of course deflated after I had both my children. I didn't notice any other unusual changes. I remember my breasts leaking about a month before with my first baby, but only after birth with my second child.

~ Sam, Northfields

When my milk 'came in' about three days after my little man was born, I had what only can be described as two massive burning squares attached to my chest. It was horrendous. I couldn't leave the house and my partner was also completely knackered, so after having read that putting cabbage leaves on your swollen lady lumps was a good source of relief, I enlisted my dad to pick some up. When he arrived at the house he produced some of Asda's finest shredded cabbage!

~ Sarah, Larne

Getting the right support—choosing a maternity bra

As pregnancy progresses your breasts will grow and grow, so unless you invest in new bras, your cups really will runneth over!

You'll probably start to outgrow your old bra sometime between eight and ten weeks. Let this be your signal to get some proper support.

Wisps of lace won't cut it anymore. Instead, invest in a well-fitting maternity or sports bra to keep your cleavage comfortable.

What do I need to look for in a maternity bra?

- **Fit:** If you can, get measured and fitted at a department store or lingerie shop. When underwear fits properly it's able to do a better job. The cups should be snug with no gaping. The centre panel should lie flat against your chest and there shouldn't be any bulgy bits over the top. Don't forget that your breasts will continue to develop and grow, so it's a good idea to get re-measured every couple of months.
- **Support:** Wide straps, supportive sides and a thick under-bust band will provide the support you need without digging into your shoulders or ribcage.
- **Coverage:** When you're choosing a maternity bra, you need to look for substance over style. Make sure the breasts are properly covered, half-cups and plunges will not provide the comfort your sensitive boobs need.
- **Growing room**: When you first buy, make sure your bra fits on the tightest fastening so there's plenty of room for growth. Lots of hook positions will ensure you can adjust it as your body changes. However, if you're getting fitted towards the end of your pregnancy, buy a bra that fastens on the loosest setting. After the birth, your ribcage will start to shrink.
- **Comfort**: Soft, breathable fabrics will feel fabulous against your skin and prevent soreness and irritation.
- **Wire worries?** Lots of expectant mums tell me they worry about wearing underwires in pregnancy. The truth is there's no evidence that underwired bras cause any harm at all, although some women find they can dig in painfully. Choose the most comfortable bra for you, whether it's wired or soft-cup.

Stop the bounce

Exercise in pregnancy can improve your fitness and keep you healthy. But your breasts will have grown and may feel tender and sore, so they will not thank you for being bounced around without the right support. Sports bras with wide, stretchy straps provide excellent lift and prevent any painful movement. They can also be useful for wearing when you're not exercising.

Sleep snug

If your breasts are particularly painful or large, you may find that wearing a bra while sleeping keeps you secure. Try a sleep bra, or look for vests or camis with 'secret support' for comfort without constriction.

Drink up

Water retention will increase hormonal swelling and soreness. Sip water to stay hydrated and beat the bloat.

Ease the itch

A combination of your skin stretching and the increased oestrogen in your blood can make your boobs ferociously itchy. Try adding bicarbonate of soda or oatmeal to your bathwater to soothe your skin.

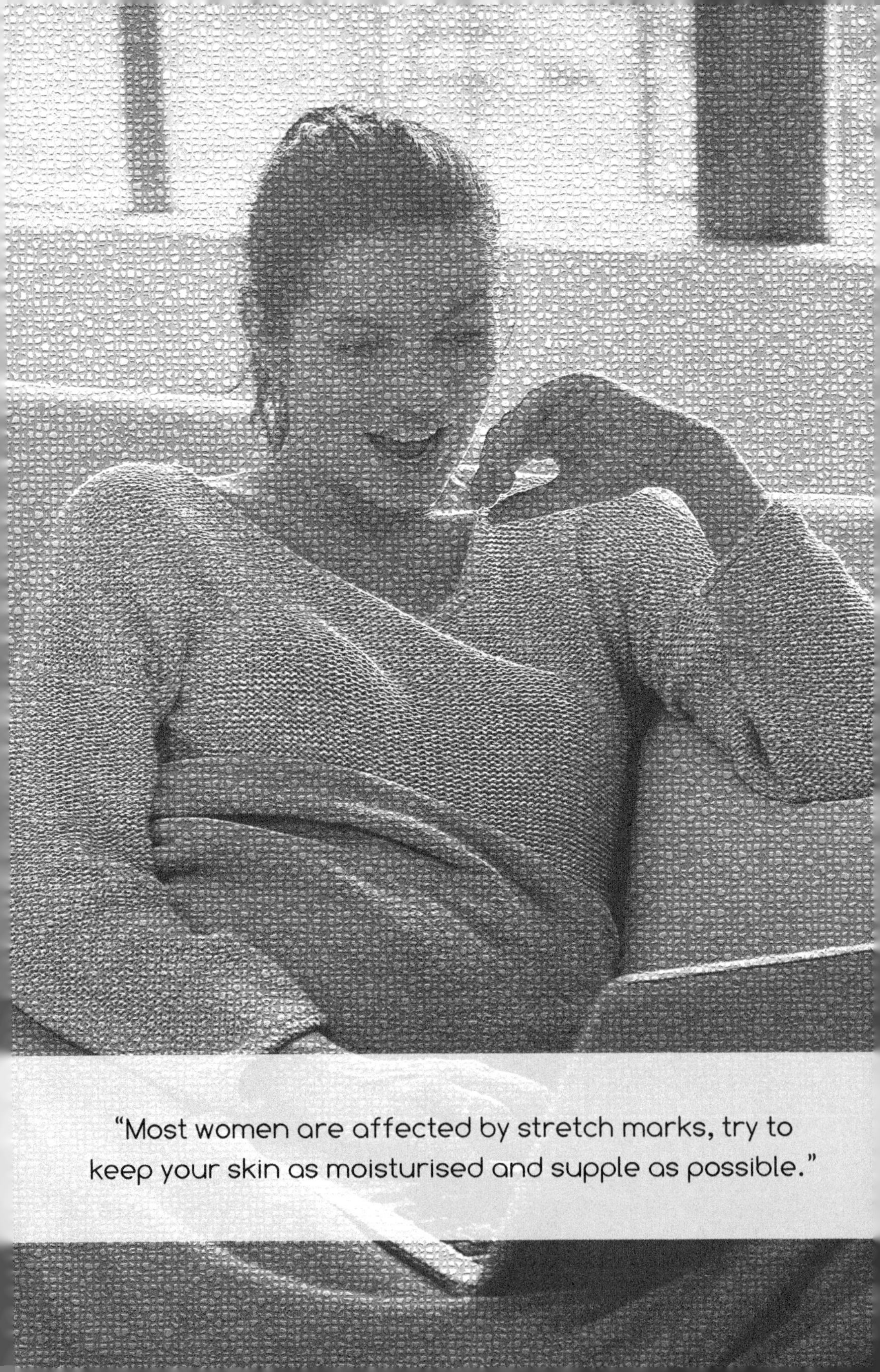

"Most women are affected by stretch marks, try to keep your skin as moisturised and supple as possible."

30

WHAT CAN I DO TO PREVENT STRETCHMARKS?

The changing body shape, rapidly expanding bump and the hormones raging around conspire to ensure that loads of women get stretch marks during pregnancy. They seem to appear overnight; you may feel a little itchy, your skin can look thin and the next minute you're covered in red stripes.

When your skin is stretched harder and faster than it can deal with, your tissues can tear, leaving a little linear wound and the purple or red streak of a stretch mark. They classically appear across the lower abdomen but can also affect your breasts, thighs and back.

They look red, angry and frankly alarming at the beginning, but with time they will fade to fine silvery lines that are barely noticeable.

Why me?

Stretch marks or **striae gravidarum** to use their scientific name, are common. In fact, by the end of pregnancy most women are affected. You're more likely to get them if they run in your family, so ask your mum if she was affected. They're also more common in darker skins, in people who gain lots of weight during pregnancy or if you're having a multiple birth.

The trouble is, once you've got them, there's little that can be done to blitz them. Although they shrink and fade with time, they don't disappear. Laser treatment or resurfacing treatments are used to help fade the colour and improve the appearance, but the elastin in the skin remains damaged and the wound is still there. Prevention is better than cure, but what can you do?

Nourish your skin

Avoid excess rapid weight gain by maintaining a healthy balanced diet and make sure you get plenty of zinc, vitamin C and vitamin E to keep your skin healthy.

Keep your skin supple:

I got terrible stretchmarks in puberty. They're all over my boobs, my thighs, my bum and even my calves. I've kind of learned to live with them, but I was paranoid about getting them in pregnancy too—it seemed like my tummy and my face were the only places without the damned things!

I was OBSESSIVE. Seriously, I rubbed oils in religiously twice a day. Some were expensive but actually, with a body oil a little goes a long way so it didn't break the bank. Anyway, I didn't get any new ones at all. I don't know if it was the oils, but I do know that my skin is prone to them and that something made a difference.

~ Elizabeth, Wetherby

Some early studies suggested that ANY cream regularly massaged into the abdomen, thighs and breasts could help to prevent stretchmarks appearing. The extra moisture and the process of massage may help the skin to stretch and adapt to your changing shape. More recent research shows that anointing your bump in cocoa butter or olive oil doesn't seem to make a blind bit of difference when it comes to stretch marks. However, regular moisturising will help make your skin soft, supple and smooth—so it's worth a try. There's no need to invest in pricey products; choose something that you like the smell and texture of and that doesn't irritate your skin. Try to make moisturising your bump and breasts part of your morning and evening routine.

Follow the evidence: I've been through the research on stretchmark treatments and I'm not going to lie, it's a little disappointing. However, the British Journal of Dermatology reported that there was some suggestion that certain lotions and potions may help prevent them appearing, so look out for these ingredients:

Centella (gotu kola or Indian pennywort) and vitamin E: Creams containing this herbal remedy together with vitamin E, appeared to protect women who developed stretchmarks in puberty from getting more during pregnancy. Gotu kola is an active herb and should not be taken orally during pregnancy. Its safety topically is less clear, so it's sensible to chat to your doctor or midwife before using it.

One mum, who was also a complementary therapist told me that she found vitamin E cream helped her stretch marks fade quicker, so it may offer some benefit.

Bitter almond oil: Massage with this oil may prevent stretchmarks appearing or reduce their severity.

Hyaluronic acid: The evidence for this working is a little weak, but hey, that's better than nothing.

After they've appeared

At the moment, there's no proven way of totally getting rid of stretch marks, and lots of mums find they can really affect their body image and sense of self-worth after the birth. While you're waiting for them to fade, if your skin is pale, a good fake tan can even out your skin colour, camouflage the stripes and boost your confidence. Pulsed dye laser therapy can be used in private clinics to fade discolouration and make the marks less conspicuous.

I was also interested to read about a new treatment developed by a team from the University of Manchester harnessing the calming properties of green tea. You don't drink it or bathe in it. Instead, it's formulated into a lotion, which has recently been launched. It is designed to tackle the marks as they appear and research is still in the early days, so watch this space.

31

WILL SEX HURT THE BABY?

It was probably sex that got you into this position in the first place—and the good news is that it's usually perfectly safe to continue enjoying sex during pregnancy. Size doesn't matter. There's no way your partner's penis can get any further than your vagina, so your baby will be safe from harm and unaware of what's happening. Your unborn child is enclosed in a bag of fluid to protect them from any bumps and bangs and there is a mucous plug safely sealing the cervix and stopping infection getting in.

Different desires

Just because sex is safe, there's no guarantee you or your partner will have the same sexual drive as you had before conception. You may find you're too tired, weak and sick to muster the energy. Your partner may find it difficult to adjust to your changing body, or may be stressed about the responsibilities of fatherhood and worried about hurting you or harming the baby. This is normal. Try not to worry, but do talk openly about it with your partner so neither of you feels hurt or rejected.

When sex isn't sensible

Sometimes sex may pose a risk to your pregnancy. Your doctor or midwife may advise you to abstain if you've had any episodes of heavy bleeding. In the first trimester, if you've had a threatened miscarriage, semen can soften the cervix and trigger cramps that could increase the risk of losing the baby. Later in pregnancy, sex may increase the risk of further bleeding if you have a low-lying placenta or if there has been bleeding behind the placenta.

If your waters have broken, it is often sensible to avoid sex because it can increase the risk of infection affecting your baby. Chat to your midwife for advice and guidance.

How will it feel?

Sex is different for all couples. Some feel highly aroused and find intercourse enjoyable, while others are happier getting a good night's sleep. It's entirely up to the two of you, but don't forget that there are lots of other ways of being intimate and making love without penetration.

Perfect positions

Your body has changed. It's tricky to get comfortable and you're probably not as agile as you used to be. So it may come as no surprise that sometimes sex can be a little awkward. It can help to explore different positions and experiment with what works for you.

Kicking off contractions

Women at the end of pregnancy and desperate for delivery often resort to the old wives' remedies of curries, castor oil and sex. The first two could be more likely to leave you crampy, bilious and uncomfortable, but sex may make a difference.

Semen contains chemicals called prostaglandins that can soften the cervix and make it ready to open up. In late pregnancy, sex or an orgasm can start off Braxton Hicks contractions, helping the womb prepare itself for labour. If this happens to you, don't panic. Try relaxing, breathing through the pain or having a warm bath until the contractions fade.

I asked a member of the Your Pregnancy Doctor team for their expert advice on sex and relationships in pregnancy. Doctor Jane has worked as an agony aunt for over twenty years:

Sex in pregnancy—positions to try

Sex in pregnancy can be intimate and enjoyable, but with that big bump getting in the way it can also be a little awkward. Let's face it, you're probably not as agile as you were, so swinging from the chandeliers is probably not on the cards. However, there are lots of positions that can allow you to enjoy each other's bodies from as early as nine days right up to nine months.

No more missionary?

The missionary position can be tricky when you're heavily pregnant. That bump gets right in the way and lying flat on your back can decrease the blood supply back to your heart making you feel dizzy, weak and faint. Not the best situation when you're trying to get in the mood. Don't worry though, you can pop a pillow under your hips to tilt your pelvis up, improving blood flow and penetration. It's a win, win situation. If that doesn't get you going, try mixing things up a little. With a little imagination, you'll find the position that really hits the spot.

Sexy spooning

Spooning can feel close and comfortable. Lie on your side with your partner lying directly behind you with their arms around you. If you find penetration difficult, don't worry, it tends to be a little shallower when you spoon. Try raising one knee towards your bump and use pillows to support your body as pregnancy progresses.

Girl on top

Being on top can take the pressure off your bump and allow you to control the depth and angle of penetration for maximum comfort and enjoyment.

Take it to the edge

Try lying or sitting on the edge of the bed while your partner stands or kneels in front of you.

Side by side

This can be one of the most successful positions in later pregnancy. You both lie at an angle to each other, using pillows to support your back and keep you comfortable. Hook both your legs over his hip, so your torsos make a v-shape. Your partner can enter you from underneath and keep his weight off your bump.

Doggy style

Sex when you're on all fours with your partner entering you from behind can be great for sexual pleasure and hitting the g-spot. However, this position definitely allows for deeper penetration, which can be uncomfortable in pregnancy. Ask your partner to be gentle and take care.

Chair flair

Try sex when your partner is sitting in a chair (choose a solid and sturdy one; you don't want to have to face complicated explanations in the emergency room). You can sit on his lap, facing him. It means you can alter the penetration and the pace to suit your needs but, be warned, it can get a little difficult when your bump gets bigger.

Mum's conundrum

I don't want my husband at the birth. In fact, I've already asked my best friend to be my birth partner. She's had two babies and I think she'll be a great support. I haven't told my husband because I don't want to hurt him. But I don't want him to see me giving birth in case it puts him off sex.

~ Anonymous, Yorkshire

Dr Jane says:

Research shows that women often have better and less traumatic births when they have an experienced female with them as well as their midwife, so your friend could really help you in labour. But you really need to talk to your husband about this. It's his baby too; what are his expectations and wishes? It's unfair to totally plan your birth without consulting him or telling him what's going on.

If he wants to be there too, many hospitals will be happy for you to have two birth partners. If you have a long labour your friend and husband may be grateful there's someone there to help take the strain so they can get some rest or have a bite to eat.

I understand your worries about your husband witnessing the delivery but there are ways of being there without seeing the gory details. Perhaps he could step outside when you start to push, or maybe he could stay at the head end. Whatever you decide, remember that a sexual relationship is not just to do with how he sees your anatomy it's also about how much you love and trust each other.

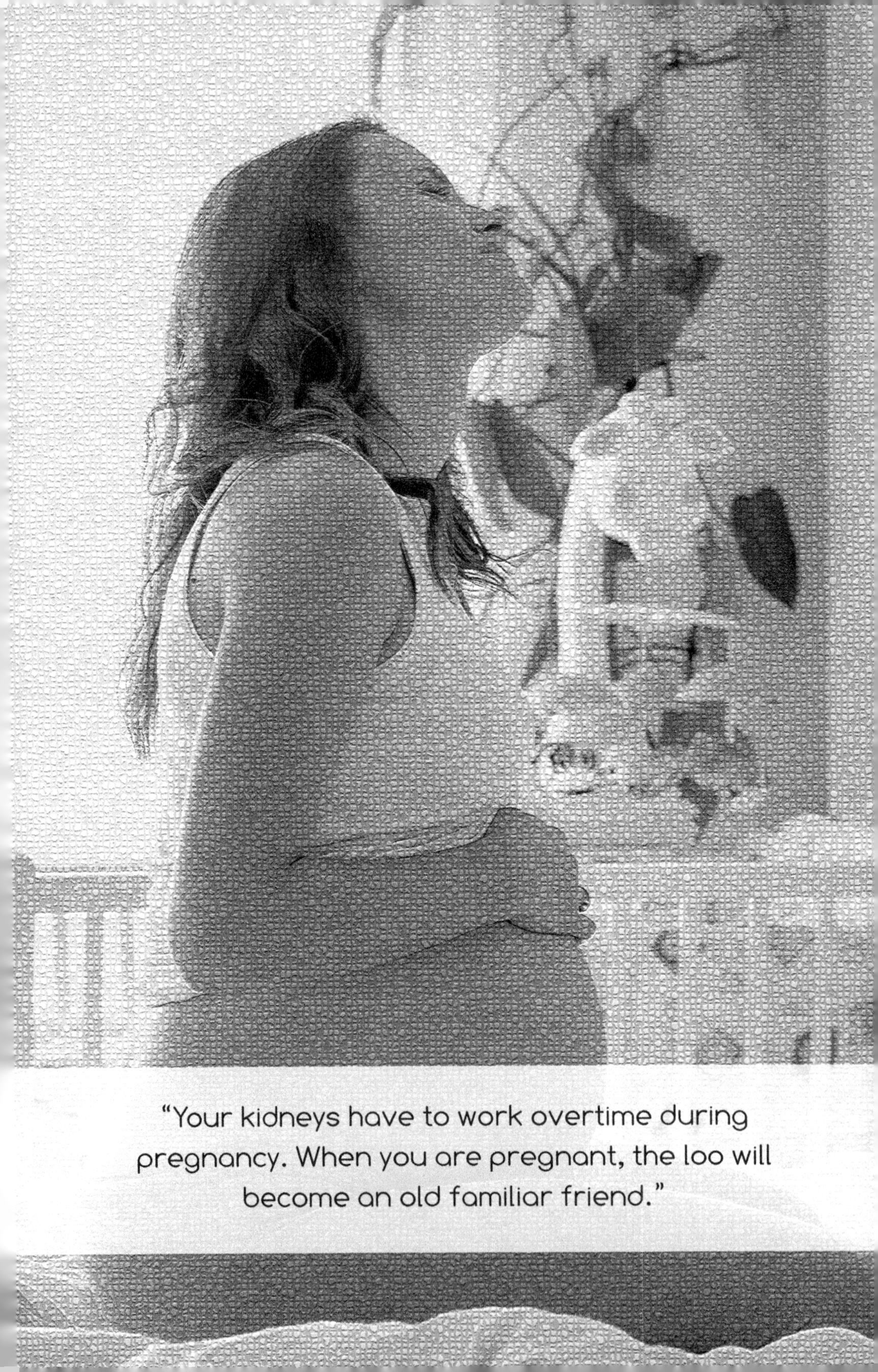

"Your kidneys have to work overtime during pregnancy. When you are pregnant, the loo will become an old familiar friend."

32

WHY AM I ALWAYS IN THE LOO?

If weeing too much is your worry, I can assure you that you're not alone. When you're pregnant, the loo will become an old, familiar friend. From as early as six weeks you may start to pee more often, and by the time your baby is due, you could be up all night trekking back and forth to the bathroom.

What's normal?

A need to pass urine more frequently during day and night can be totally normal. As with many of pregnancy's irritations, it's down to hormones and increased circulating blood. Your kidneys have to work overtime, which means there's more waste to flush. Later, your expanding womb presses against your bladder making ever more frequent trips to the loo essential. To compound this, if you have puffy ankles, the fluid will be absorbed back into your bloodstream while you're asleep, making an unbroken night's sleep a thing of the past.

What's not?

Sometimes passing urine too often can signal danger:

- **Urine infections**: Pregnant women are more prone to cystitis. Burning or stinging when you pass water, the presence of blood, feeling feverish and unwell, or developing an aching pain in your loins could indicate an infection.

  Urine infections can be more serious in pregnancy, so even if you're used to cystitis, don't just watch and wait. Take a sample to your doctor's surgery as soon as you can. It is important to treat UTIs promptly in pregnancy to prevent the infection spreading to the kidneys or the blood stream, or triggering premature labour. So it's a good idea to check with your GP before using over-the-counter treatments.

- **Gestational diabetes**: If you develop pregnancy diabetes you may notice that you need to wee a lot, even more than the normal pregnancy frequency. You may also have a dry mouth and a raging thirst which can't be quenched by drinking lots. Many women feel increasingly lethargic, have repeated infections like thrush and their vision may become blurry or unclear. Many people will be diagnosed as having gestational diabetes before they become unwell or notice any significant symptoms, but if you're worried, see your doctor promptly.

Protect yourself

There are ways to stave off cystitis, prevent infections and keep your bladder healthy in pregnancy:

- **Stay hydrated**: Too many women don't drink enough because they're worried about getting to the loo. But dehydration can irritate your bladder and increase the risk of infection. Plenty of fluids will ensure your bladder is flushed regularly.

- **Listen to your body**: Don't cross your legs and hold on! Pass urine when you need to.
- **Empty your bladder**: Your expanding uterus can make it difficult to fully empty your bladder, which means it'll fill up more quickly next time. Try leaning forward when you wee and rocking backwards and forwards to help empty the bladder more efficiently. It can also be a good idea to try to go again when you think you've finished, to get rid of any late drips.
- **Safe sex**: Sex can increase the risk of infection, so pee before and after intercourse to prevent cystitis.
- **Careful cleaning**: Women are at greater risk of infection because the urinary opening is pretty close to the anus, so it's easy for bacteria to get into the bladder and cause infection. Good toilet hygiene can prevent that happening. Wipe carefully after going to the loo, going from front to back. I know that can be tricky when you're negotiating a big bump, but it is much safer for you and your baby.
- Slurp down some cranberry juice; it can help fight off infection.

Controlling the urge

Some things will increase your need to wee, you can reduce your time on the loo by:

- Cutting out caffeinated drinks like cola, coffee and tea (they have a diuretic effect)
- Making sure your bladder is empty before you go to bed
- Avoiding drinks immediately before bedtime
- Decreasing your ankle swelling by putting your feet up in the evenings to allow fluid to drain away

Testing your urine

At each and every antenatal appointment, from the day of booking through to the day of delivery, you'll be asked to give a urine specimen. Your urine can tell us an awful lot about your health. It will usually be tested using a special dipstick that can immediately detect specific substances that could indicate disease.

Your urine is screened for the presence of glucose or sugar, protein and blood. And although small amounts of both glucose and protein are normally present in urine, high levels can indicate a problem, which may require further testing and investigation.

Protein

A high level of protein in the urine may indicate a number of things. You're tested regularly to ensure you don't develop kidney problems or pre-eclampsia, a serious pregnancy complication in which your kidneys leak protein. This can happen in combination with increased swelling of the body and your blood pressure becoming dangerously high.

However, if you spot, a + or two in your antenatal notes, don't panic. Your protein level could be raised because of urine infection, due to the effect of some medication or simply due to contamination from a little vaginal discharge or a dirty urine pot, so don't let one abnormal dipstick stress you out.

Your midwife or doctor will check your blood pressure, send your urine off to test for an infection and may arrange for repeat screening.

Glucose

I was so stressed when my urine showed loads of glucose, it was +++ or something like that. I felt totally fine and I was really worried about gestational diabetes. The next test was normal, which was weird. In the end, it was incredibly embarrassing because I'd saved my sample in an old honey jar, that I hadn't washed out properly! I used the proper containers from then on.

~ Louise, York

High urine glucose levels may be a sign that either you already had undiagnosed type 2 diabetes before you became pregnant, or you have recently developed gestational diabetes, a form of diabetes that can develop during pregnancy.

A little glucose doesn't mean that you've definitely got diabetes. In fact, around half of all women will get a positive dipstick at some stage, because the kidneys can tend to leak a little sugar during pregnancy. If you get a positive urine test, you will usually have a follow-up blood glucose test, and maybe a special glucose tolerance test to check how well your body is able to deal with sugar and other carbohydrates.

Blood

Your urine will be routinely tested for haemoglobin. A little blood can be present without any change in colour. Blood can indicate an early infection, even if you don't have any pain or problems passing urine. It's important to catch these early because urinary tract infections can spread to your kidneys and into your bloodstream, putting you at risk of severe illness and kidney damage, and also potentially triggering miscarriage and premature labour.

However, there could be a little blood from your vagina if you've had bleeding or a show. Your urine will be sent away for further analysis.

Ketones

Ketones are chemicals produced by the body when it burns fat for energy. It can happen when you're not eating enough because of nausea and vomiting, especially if you are suffering from hyperemesis gravidarum. If this is the case, you may need to be admitted to hospital for treatment and rehydration with a drip.

If ketones are found together with sugar, this could be a sign of diabetic ketoacidosis, a dangerous complication of diabetes, which would also require admission and fluids and insulin treatment for a while to get things under control.

Laboratory analysis

If you have any symptoms of infection, or your urine is showing blood and protein, you may have a UTI. Your doctor or midwife will ask for a sample of your urine to send off for testing. This should be from the middle of your urine stream, so wee a bit, catch some, then empty your bladder. The lab will look at the urine, see if any bugs grow and check the best antibiotics to blitz them.

33

ISN'T THE STRESS OF MY STOPPING SMOKING WORSE FOR MY BABY THAN THE FUMES?

This is one of the things that lots of mums say to me in an attempt to justify continuing to smoke. I understand—it's tough to give up cigarettes. Nicotine's an addictive drug and smoking can be a seductive habit that can draw you back in, even when you're desperate to quit.

You may think that smoking calms and relaxes you, but your body is getting a whole different experience. In fact, each puff of smoke speeds up your heart and bumps up your blood pressure. That's what happens with stress too, except with stress you're not getting 4,000 toxic chemicals as well!

In making the decision to light up when you're pregnant, it's important to understand the harm that tobacco can do to your pregnancy and your unborn child, and that means knowing the difference between the facts and the falsehoods. These are the other comments I hear in my consulting room:

I'm past the first trimester, so it's too late now

The sooner you quit, the better. But believe me, it's never too late. As soon as you stop smoking, your baby's body will notice the difference. As your lungs clear the smoke, the carbon monoxide levels in your body will fall and your oxygen levels will return to normal. Rapidly, the oxygen flow through the placenta will increase, which will improve your baby's health and wellbeing, whatever stage of pregnancy you're at.

If my baby's small, I'll have an easy birth

I've heard this many times; small babies are cute and slip out more easily. Yes, babies of all sizes are gorgeous, but sadly babies whose growth has been stunted by cigarette smoke are less healthy. Low birth weight isn't just about size. Being born small is also associated with higher risks of chest infections and asthma as well as death in early infancy. It's a serious matter.

My mum smoked and drank throughout labour and I came out OK

In the past women were definitely less careful in pregnancy. But we know that smoking can cause problems with pregnancy because we've researched the impact on past pregnancies and come out with cold, hard statistics. It's a matter of risk; smoking does increase the risk of miscarriage, stillbirth and low birth weight. However, that doesn't mean that lots of babies aren't born perfectly healthy. It's a roll of the dice—are you happy to gamble on your baby?

I'll gain weight if I stop, and that's worse for my baby

It's true that too much weight gain can predispose to gestational diabetes and pregnancy problems. However, the risks with smoking are significantly greater. But how about quitting and NOT gaining loads of weight? With clearer lungs, you'll feel more fit, so you can do more exercise and by binning the booze in pregnancy, there'll be fewer empty calories, so you can maintain a healthy pregnancy weight gain, without piling on the pounds.

I can't quit, so there's no point in cutting down

I know it's hard to kick the habit. Up to five per cent of mums continue to smoke in pregnancy, and although a number of studies have tried to get them to stop, they don't.

Although there is no safe level of smoking, the damaging effects of smoking are thought to be dose-related, so it's better to cut down than do nothing. If you're on twenty a day and say you can't quit, why don't you have those you find the hardest to give up? When you wake up in the morning you can have a cigarette if you have to, but don't have another until your mid-morning cup of tea. At lunchtime after your meal, have one more cigarette.

That means you have had three cigarettes. Then you can say, 'Well, I'm going to see how long I can go without a cigarette.' The hardest one will be after your evening meal and the one before you go to bed, so try to hold out for these.

This means you are only having five cigarettes a day. It's not ideal, but it is significantly preferable to smoking an entire packet. Your baby will thank you for it.

Top ten reasons to quit smoking during pregnancy

Are you struggling to find the motivation to give up smoking? Quitting can be the greatest single thing you do for your body and for your baby, and here's why:

- **You'll have a healthier new born baby**
  It's a frightening fact that babies are 33% more likely to be stillborn, or to sadly die within the first week if they are born to smokers.

- **You'll prevent cot death**
  Sudden infant death syndrome is a devastating condition. Smoking trebles the risk of cot death in your baby. Is that enough reason to quit?

- **Think of the money you'll save**
  Let's face it, fags are horrendously expensive—and let me let you in on a secret, babies are too. Instead of setting fire to your cash, save it in a big glass jar. Then have a splurge—you'll definitely deserve it.

- **You'll be kissable any time, any place, anywhere**
  With no fag to puff, your breath will be minty fresh, so you can enjoy a spontaneous snog any time of the day of night, with no fear of halitosis.

- **Your skin will look younger for longer**
  Smoking makes you age quicker. The toxic chemicals damage the delicate collagen and elastin in the skin, leaving it prematurely saggy and wrinkly.

- **You'll smell fresh and fabulous**
  Take a sniff of some of your old, unwashed smoky clothes. That's what you smell like to a non-smoker. It's not exactly appealing is it? If you quit, that eau de ashtray scent will be a thing of the past.

- **No more shivering outside restaurants, cafes or your workplace**
  The government have made it a lot less comfortable to smoke. Now you have to huddle under porches and umbrellas to get a puff. Is that what you want when you're out and about with your baby?

- **You'll stay healthy for longer**
  It's not just about you anymore. Soon you will be part of a family, with a baby depending on you for care, comfort and love. The sad truth is that cigarette smoking causes premature death, with smokers living on average ten years less than non-smokers. By quitting, you can cut the risk, and help ensure your little one has a healthy mum for longer.

- **You'll protect your unborn child**
  Babies born to women who smoke are on average 200g or eight ounces lighter than babies born to non-smoking mothers. And the frightening truth is that the more cigarettes a woman smokes during pregnancy, the greater the reduction in the baby's birth weight.

  When you smoke, your baby does too. The nicotine, poisonous chemicals and carbon monoxide cross the placenta into the baby's bloodstream. Research suggests that cigarettes can reduce the flow of blood in the placenta, which limits the amounts of important nutrients that reach your baby.

- **No more cringing in the doctor's surgery**
  I'm sure you've had enough of people nagging you about the perils of tobacco. Well, if you quit you won't have to hear that any more. You'll be an ex-smoker. Doesn't that feel good?

Help to quit

I understand that it can be horribly hard to quit. Don't worry, you are not alone. There are specialist midwives and stop-smoking advisors to provide support, and here are some tips to help you on your way:

A helping hand

Ask your midwife or doctor for help, support and guidance. You can be referred to a stop smoking team for specialist advice. They offer one-to-one appointments or group sessions to help you quit. The programme is typically twelve weeks but they'll respond to your individual needs and help you cope with cravings and nicotine withdrawal.

Craving-busters

Nicotine replacement therapies like patches, gum, lozenges and sprays can quell the craving for nicotine and help you give up. The nicotine isn't the worst bit of smoking for you or your baby. Carbon monoxide gas, tar and other noxious chemicals are much more dangerous. Chat to your doctor, midwife or stop-smoking adviser about the safe options in more detail. Vaping and electronic cigarettes are popular but their contents are currently not controlled so they are not recommended in pregnancy at the moment.

Believe in yourself

Try to picture yourself as an ex-smoker. It may be tricky in the early days, but remember that four out of five women who manage to stop smoking for twenty-eight days manage it for good. So take it one day at a time; you CAN do it.

Get tested

You will be offered a carbon monoxide test early in your pregnancy. Get your levels checked as a brilliant incentive to quit the weed. This poisonous gas enters the body when you smoke, meaning that your blood can carry less oxygen to your baby. Lower oxygen can slow growth, affect development, increase the risk of miscarriage and stillbirth and predispose to cot death after the birth. The test will check how high your levels are and see how much your baby could be affected.

Keep it fresh

Have a toothbrush or some gum at the ready to keep your mouth fresh and fabulous. You may be less likely to sully it with ciggies.

Think of the cash

Fags are expensive. Put the money you'd have burned into a big glass jar. You can spend it on stuff for your new baby or indulge yourself with a massage, a pedicure or a longed-for treat.

Rope in family and friends

People who quit together, stick together. Your partner or close family members can support you by stopping smoking too.

Sniff it out

Stick some of your old smoky clothes in a bag at the back of the wardrobe and have a big sniff when you're tempted to light up, it'll show you how you used to smell!

Change your routine

If you get your cigarettes from the same shop on the way to work, then change your route. If you grab a fag outside with your mates at lunchtime, try having a swim or taking a walk instead. If coffee and a cigarette has always been your breakfast, savour something fresh and nourishing like Greek yoghurt with berries. In short, try anything to break ingrained bad habits and start some new healthier ones.

It worked for us—Mums' stop smoking tips

I changed my routine. I used to have a cigarette and a coffee before setting off for work. Now `I leave a little earlier and have my breakfast with friends at the work canteen. It's fun and there's a no smoking rule, so I'm never tempted.

~ Fi, Leeds

I know you shouldn't but I told my family and close mates I was pregnant straight away. It meant that everyone was watching me, so I didn't dare smoke. They'd have nagged me stupid.

~ Hannah, Rugby

I used to get my ciggies from a newsagent on my way to the bus stop, I sort of walked in automatically every time I went past. I started going to a different bus stop instead, and it was so much easier not to be tempted.

~ Evie, Leeds

Dr Keith says:

Plan a date to quit. The week before put your cigarette butts in a jar half filled with water. When you've given up, place £5 in the jar every day and at the end of the week treat yourself. The cash should hopefully be more appealing than the butt-filled jar.

34

WHAT ARE MY MATERNITY RIGHTS AT WORK?

Different countries have different rights and restrictions, but in the UK the days of being sacked, overlooked and badly treated at work during pregnancy should be over. The United Kingdom has a set of laws that helps to protect the rights and responsibilities of pregnant women in the workplace.

As a pregnant working woman, you have rights. These allow you paid time off for essential antenatal appointments as well as leave to care for your baby and recover from the birth.

There's an awful lot of confusing leaflets, forms, facts and figures to absorb. Here's a basic overview. Chat to your employer and check-out suggested links and you can ensure you get what you are entitled to.

Paid time off for antenatal care

When I talk about antenatal care, that covers antenatal appointments, scans, tests and also antenatal or parenting classes, if they've been recommended by your doctor or midwife.

Your partner's entitled to time-off too, so they can share the joy and excitement of the scan and hear their baby's heartbeat for the first time. The father (or partner of your choice) has the right to unpaid time off work to go to two antenatal appointments.

The number of antenatal appointments usually covered is somewhere between seven and ten. However, this is flexible and if there is a valid medical reason, you may be entitled to more. This could be the case if you have gestational diabetes or placenta praevia, or if your baby needs extra monitoring.

It gets a little tricky if you don't want to tell anyone you're pregnant yet. Many women prefer to wait until after twelve weeks to share their happy news, when the risk of miscarriage drops. It's also not unusual to wait a little longer to inform work, to avoid being dealt with differently. If that's you, you'll have to rely on annual leave, or self-certified sick leave for 'doctor's appointments' to sneak away discreetly, without too many fibs or too much subterfuge.

The right to maternity leave

Every pregnant employee is entitled to up to a year of maternity leave. It doesn't matter how many hours you work, how long you've been employed or how much your salary is, you can still claim the time off, as long as you give your employer the correct notice.

It's compulsory to take two weeks off after childbirth (four weeks if you work in a factory) to care for your baby and allow your body to recuperate and recover. After that, it's up to you when you choose to return to work.

Eligible employees can take up to 52 weeks' maternity leave. The first 26 weeks is known as 'Ordinary Maternity Leave,' and the last 26 weeks as 'Additional Maternity Leave.' The earliest that leave can be taken is eleven weeks before the expected week of childbirth, unless the baby is born early.

The right to Maternity Pay or Maternity Allowance

Pregnancy can be an expensive time. For something so small, a baby can really cost a lot. But it can be a real challenge to work when you're heavily pregnant. and you'll need time off to recover from the birth and care for your baby. The good news is that if you have been working, you should be entitled to financial support during your maternity leave.

What is Statutory Maternity Pay?

If you're eligible you are entitled to a fixed weekly payment for up to 39 weeks while you're on leave. This is called Statutory Maternity Pay (SMP) and it will usually start when you go on maternity leave. However, it will also be triggered automatically if you're off work for a pregnancy-related illness in the four weeks before your baby is due.

Am I eligible?

You're entitled to SMP if you're an employed pregnant woman who has:

- Worked for your employer for at least 26 weeks by the time you reach the end of the 15th week before your baby is due. Calculate this by finding the Sunday before your due date and counting back exactly 15 weeks.
- Earned an average of at least £113 per week.

How much is SMP?

For the current 2017-18 tax year, Statutory Maternity pay is:

Start of leave to 6 weeks	90% of average weekly earnings before tax
6 weeks to 39 weeks	£140.98 or 90% of average weekly earnings, whichever is lower
39 to 52 weeks	Unpaid

Talk to your employer

Different companies offer different maternity policies; many offer enhanced maternity pay. Chat to your HR department, or whoever deals with leave and find out what happens where you work.

I had really good HR support in my work. I had issues with the guy chosen to cover my position whilst I was on maternity leave in that he was openly stating that he wouldn't go back to his old job after I returned, but the strong HR support I had made sure any concerns were put to bed.

~ Kirsty, Annalong

How do I claim?

To claim maternity leave, you need to let your employer know when you want to stop work. This should be done by the 15th week before the baby's due date, which will be when you are around 25 weeks pregnant. Calculate the exact deadline by finding the Sunday before your due date and counting back 15 weeks. Your employer must write to you within 28 days confirming your start and end dates.

You have to give your employer proof that you're pregnant to get SMP. Your doctor or midwife can provide this in the form of a letter or a MATB1 certificate. It's important to give at least 21 days' notice that you want to start SMP, or as much as possible if your baby is born early.

Maternity Allowance

Lots of women are unable to claim SMP because they're self-employed, they haven't worked in their job for long enough or because their pay is below the £113 limit. The good news is that there is still some financial support available in the form of Maternity Allowance. It's a fortnightly or monthly payment from the government, that varies depending on your earnings.

How much is Maternity Allowance?

The amount of Maternity Allowance you would receive in the 2017-18 tax year would be:

Start of leave to 39 weeks	£140.98 or 90% of average weekly earnings, whichever is lower
For up to a further 14 weeks	£27 per week

Protection against unfair treatment, discrimination or dismissal

Employers can't change a pregnant employee's contract terms and conditions without their agreement. If they do, they are in breach of contract. They also have to ensure that the work environment is safe. When the employee tells her employer she's pregnant, the employer should assess the risks to the woman and her baby.

Examples of risks include heavy lifting or carrying, exposure to toxic substances, and long working hours without breaks. Where there are risks, the employer should take reasonable steps to remove them, for example, by offering the employee different work or changing their hours. If they cannot either remove the risks or offer suitable alternative work, the employer should suspend the employee on *full pay*.

Everything was OK at work for me. I was allowed to go to the bathroom when I needed it, and could bring drinks and snacks so I could eat or drink when I needed to. I was also given the option of lighter duties.

~ Sam, Northfields

While this legislation has made life better for pregnant women in the workplace, I don't think it goes far enough. I have seen through the women I care for that pregnancy can be tough, both for women with high-powered jobs and for those doing exhausting physical work. I feel strongly that the medical profession should do more to educate employers about the risks pregnant women face.

I believe that pregnant women can, and indeed should, still go to work and pursue their normal activities, but they should have the opportunity to take an hour's rest in the morning, take their lunch break properly, and also have an hour's rest in the afternoon. Pregnant women are good at sleeping for short periods of time and waking up full of energy. It is the nature of being pregnant and employers should appreciate this. It's only through adapting that we can get the best out of the workforce, and nurture the babies who will be the future of this country.

Find out more:

www.moneyadviceservice.org.uk
www.maternityaction.org.uk
www.gov.uk/maternity-pay-leave/how-to-claim

35

WHAT CAN I DO ABOUT PELVIC PAIN?

From the beginning of pregnancy your body starts to adapt to allow the delivery of your new baby. The hormone relaxin loosens the ligaments holding the pelvis together, so it can stretch during labour. This makes birth much easier but it can also cause a few problems along the way.

Many of my patients complain about problems with agonising pelvic pain, especially towards the end of pregnancy. As many as one in five pregnant women get pelvic girdle pain when they walk, climb stairs or turn over in bed. The aches, cramps and dragging pains can be utterly miserable. The good news is that the pain won't harm your baby. and early diagnosis and treatment can help soothe the discomfort and help you stay mobile.

Pelvic girdle pain

PGP, SPD, DSP. That's a whole lot of confusing acronyms adding up to one thing. Pain. Pelvic girdle pain (PGP) is simply the new name for the condition we used to call *symphysis pubis dysfunction (SPD)*.

The weight of your growing baby and the changes in your posture in pregnancy put more strain on the pelvis. The soft, stretchy ligaments mean that the joints between the bones in the pelvis may move unevenly and the pelvic girdle can become unstable and painful. Sometimes the bones at the front of the pelvis can separate further in a condition known as *diastasis symphysis pubis*, which causes severe pain and increased difficulty moving.

If you have PGP you may experience:

- **Pain**: The pain may be in the pubic region, the hips, groin and thighs or in the lower back and knees
- **Clicking**: You may notice a clicking or grinding noise
- **Difficulty moving**: The pain may get worse if you walk on uneven surfaces, if you open your legs, if you stand on one leg or if you have sex

Who is affected?

Pelvic pain can strike any pregnant woman, particularly in the latter months. You are more likely to suffer pain if you have had back or pelvic problems in the past. It is also more likely if you have hypermobility syndrome.

> *I suffered from major pelvic pain in pregnancy, because my bump was so big, even from early on. I found my GP really unhelpful as he basically told me to put up with it. I wish I'd known where to get help.*
>
> **~ Kirsty, Annalong**

PGP can vary from mild to severe. The pain and movement restrictions can sometimes make it difficult to get on with normal life. Getting out of the car, getting dressed, even going to the loo can be a real challenge. The good news is that it is treatable and the sooner you get help, the better. You don't have to put up with it. See your doctor or midwife so they can refer you to a specialist physiotherapist for assessment, advice and support.

How to help yourself

There are a few ways to ease the pain and keep moving:

- **Listen to your body**: Get plenty of rest to take the weight off your pelvis.
- **Try to stay active**: Swimming is a wonderful activity in pregnancy, allowing you to move while the water supports your weight. However, be careful with breast-stroke, the leg and hip action may aggravate the pain.
- **Perfect posture**: Try to stand upright, tucking your bottom in.
- **On an even keel**: If you are standing still or getting up from sitting, put equal weight on both legs.
- **Mix it up**: Don't stay in one position for long periods.
- **Make life easy**: Standing on one leg is difficult, so stay seated when you get dressed or undressed.
- **Don't spread your legs**: If you can, keep your knees together when getting in or out of the car. Ask your partner to lend a hand if you're struggling.
- **Sleep easy**: Use a pillow between your legs and under your bump for extra support and comfort.
- **Avoid triggers**: Lifting, twisting, crossing your legs and climbing stairs can make the pain worse. Be sensible and take life easy whenever you can.
- **Take pain relief**: Regular paracetamol can calm pain and is thought to be safe when taken according to the instructions.

Expert help

Although you can make a difference yourself, if your pain is severe you'll need support and treatment. A specialist physiotherapist, osteopath or chiropractor can be a fantastic source of guidance and expertise. They may suggest:

- Good postural positions and ways to avoid pain
- Exercises to improve balance, core strength and stability
- Hands-on therapy to mobilise the joints
- Hot and cold compresses to relieve inflammation or muscle spasm
- Hydrotherapy to soothe and support
- Acupuncture: this ancient Chinese therapy uses fine needles inserted at specific points in the body to restore any imbalance in energy or qi and relieve pain
- A wide stretchy belt to support your bump and help stabilise your pelvis
- Crutches if you are struggling with mobility

Birth and beyond

The idea of labour when you struggle to even open your knees can be terrifying. But I can assure you that most women with pelvic pain in pregnancy are able to have a normal vaginal birth. Talk to your healthcare team about the best pain relief options for you; there are lots of choices, including an epidural. Alternatively, consider a birth pool. The water will support your body so you can move more freely during labour.

The pain usually settles after birth, although ten per cent of women may have ongoing problems. If that's you, continue using pain relief and seeing the physio until the pain goes away and you're moving normally.

36

IS IT SAFE TO INDULGE MY CRAVINGS?

If you went by what you see in films, you'd assume that all pregnant women are nipping to their local store late at night to stock up on pickled onions and ice-cream. But many women don't experience any unusual cravings. If you do, as long as it's part of a healthy, balanced diet, it's fine to indulge. But if you're eyeing up the coal scuttle hungrily, it's time to see your doctor. Pica is the name for the craving for non-edible items, like coal, petrol, baking soda, sand and even broken china. It's important not to give into these desires. They could harm you and the baby, and they could also be a sign of nutritional deficiencies and anaemia.

Constant cravings?

Fancy a banana and marmite sandwich, ice-cream with a side of mustard or even a little coal and mud? Your pregnant body can play all sorts of tricks on your tastebuds, going off old favourites and longing for something more eccentric.

Your cravings may run the gamut from cheeseburgers to chalk. Believe me, I've cared for women who've longed for everything from strawberries to soil. Research shows us that somewhere between fifty and ninety per cent of American women crave specific foods in pregnancy. They usually start towards the end of the first trimester, tempt the taste-buds throughout the middle months and tend to tail off in the last trimester and drop off dramatically following delivery.

A study demonstrated that women commonly craved sweet stuff: ice cream, fruit juice, sweets, desserts, dairy, and chocolate were popular, as was fresh fruit. Longings for salty or savoury foods were less common, although some studies do demonstrate cravings for curries and pizza. Hmmm... maybe I'm pregnant too!

Mums confess their pregnancy cravings

I craved malted milk biscuits with number one right up to the day I went into hospital and with number two I loved the smell of tarmac—I didn't eat it though!

~ Amanda, Chichester

Having always been a healthy eater and conscious of diet, I was horrified when I started craving McDonald's meals! I had to limit myself to the number I ate and continued with a healthy low GI diet, but it was definitely a guilty pleasure.

~ Chloe, Guildford

I loved the mix of sweet and savoury in pregnancy, so banana and Marmite or jam and cheese on toast were real favourites. I have to be honest though, I still like those combinations and my kids are both at school now!

~ Jane, Leeds

A good excuse?

Let's face it, we all fancy certain foods every now and then. Whether it's salted caramel ice-cream, peanuts or cheesecake, some foods can really get our juices flowing. Most of us try to suppress those urges because eating everything we fancy whenever we fancy it instead of choosing a balanced nutritious diet is likely to leave us fat and sluggish. Could it be that pregnancy is used as an excuse to indulge? When you're expecting, it's cute and socially acceptable to send your partner to the shops at midnight to get your favourite treat.

I'm not saying it's all about greed, but maybe some cravings are about fancying foods rather than irresistible urges.

Gestational diabetes

Women who are obese, with a BMI of over 30, have a higher risk of developing gestational diabetes. It's also more likely if you pile on the pounds during pregnancy. And your weight won't just affect you, a baby born to an obese mother is at higher risk of stillbirth and congenital abnormalities as well as obesity and type 2 diabetes in the future. So it's clear that you shouldn't give in to your cravings unless they're for lean meat and vegetables!

Pica problems

Top seven non-food cravings

- Ice
- Coal
- Toothpaste
- Sponge (that's the bath-type not the jam and buttercream variety)
- Mud
- Chalk
- Laundry soap

Survey by Gurgle.com

It's not fully understood why some women develop pica. However, many doctors believe that it may be the way our bodies show that we need important minerals. This seems to be confirmed by research, with studies showing that women who developed pica during pregnancy were more likely to be deficient in iron. Many expectant mums crave ice. This could be because it soothes a sore tongue, which is common with anaemia. Ice is pretty harmless but swigging petrol or chowing down on chalk and soil clearly isn't!

If you are getting a totally balanced diet with the micronutrients you need, it's likely you won't suffer any strong or dangerous cravings. If you're struggling to control your cravings, try a multivitamin supplement designed for pregnant women and see your doctor for support and guidance.

37

IS THE POSITION OF THE PLACENTA IMPORTANT?

The placenta is your baby's lifeline, linking them to you and a ready flow of oxygen, energy and nutrition. It develops wherever your fertilised egg embeds in your womb. This can be anywhere; the front, the back, the top or the sides are totally normal. The placental position is important because it can sometimes cause problems later on in pregnancy and during the birth.

What's where?

The position of the placenta is usually located during your routine scan between 18 and 21 weeks. At this stage, the position will be described as one of the following:

- **Anterior**: on the front wall of your womb
- **Posterior**: on the back of the uterus
- **Fundal**: in the top wall of the womb
- **Lateral**: on the side of the uterus and described as right or left lateral

The placenta may also be identified as being in the lower part of the womb, which if it stays there to the end of pregnancy is known as **placenta praevia**.

Anterior placenta

If the placenta develops on the front wall of the womb, it is usually not a big problem. However, in the second trimester, you may find it prevents you from feeling your baby's early movements. Your little one may be kicking like crazy and turning somersaults in there, but you may not feel it because the placenta cushions you from the action. You may feel the first flutters a little later and also the movement may seem muted until the later stages of pregnancy when their little legs and muscles have developed and they can kick hard enough to make their presence felt.

An anterior placenta can cause difficulties if you need a Caesarean section, simply because it can get in the way. There could also be an increased risk of bleeding because the placenta may lie exactly where your obstetrician needs make their incision. To prevent problems, I usually do a later scan so I know precisely where the placenta lies and I can plan exactly where I'll cut into the womb. Sometimes it's necessary to make the incision a little higher to minimise the risk of blood loss.

Placenta praevia

A placenta praevia lies low in the womb. It can affect as many as one in two hundred pregnancies. Placenta praevia is more common in mums who are a little older as well as in women who have had a Caesarean section or another low-lying placenta in the past.

When the placenta lies low, it can block the neck of the womb, or it may overlap it slightly. It can cause bleeding in the last trimester and if it stays in position over the cervix, a vaginal delivery could put the mother at risk of a severe haemorrhage. In this case, a Caesarean section is needed to protect mum and baby.

How is it picked up?

A low placenta is usually identified during the routine anomaly scan. At this stage, a low placenta is relatively common. The position often changes in the last few months, as the baby's head engages and stretches the lower part of the uterus. The greater expansion of lower part of the womb often moves the placenta further away from the neck of the womb.

My first scan showed that my placenta was low, but I was reassured it would probably move out of the way later in pregnancy. At thirty weeks, I started bleeding. It was like a heavy period, and I was rushed into hospital. I had to stay there for a week, lying in bed, until things totally stopped. It was very frightening and it seemed certain I would have to have a Caesarean because the placenta was blocking the way. I was amazed when my thirty-six-week scan showed the placenta had moved and I am now planning a normal delivery.

~ Michelle, London

If your placenta is identified as being low, you'll be given an extra ultrasound scan later in your pregnancy, usually at about 32 weeks. The sonographer will recheck the position of the placenta, the good news is that as many as 90% will have moved away from the cervix by this stage, so pregnancy and labour can carry on as normal.

However, if the placenta still lies low it can block the neck of the womb (major placenta praevia) or overlap it slightly (minor placenta praevia). This gets right in the way of your baby's entrance into the world. There is a significant chance of bleeding (both in pregnancy and during the birth) which could put you and your baby at risk. In this case, a Caesarean section is needed to protect mum and baby.

Staying safe

Placenta praevia can cause heavy, painless vaginal bleeding, usually in the last months of pregnancy. If you experience bleeding, it's vital to get medical help urgently. A scan may be done to see if an emergency Caesarean is needed, and sometimes women need bed rest or hospital admission for the rest of their pregnancy. This is so a section or emergency treatment such as transfusions can be carried out quickly and efficiently.

If your placenta is covering the cervix and you have bled, you will probably be admitted to hospital from approximately 34 weeks of gestation. If you've had no problems or have minor praevia, you may be able to stay at home. However, it's important to have safety measures in place, in case of emergency.

- Have someone available to help twenty-four hours a day
- Have ready access to the hospital
- Know that you should attend immediately if you have bleeding, contractions or pain

If this sounds scary, I'm sorry. I don't want to frighten you, just let you know the possible risks. I can tell you that there is also excellent news. Most babies whose mums had low lying placentas are born healthily and with no complications.

In this section, I also want to talk about two other placental problems. Although these conditions aren't related to placental position, they are serious disorders I want to bring to your attention so you know when to get medical help:

Placental abruption

If the name placental abruption sounds rather sudden and scary, that's because it is.

It describes a condition where part of the placenta tears away from the womb, while the baby is still in the womb. An abruption of the placenta can have serious consequences for you and your baby. It affects as many as one in a hundred pregnancies, so it's a good idea to be aware of the symptoms and signs.

Blood and tears

The placenta is richly supplied with blood, which means even a small tear can lead to heavy bleeding. The blood may leak out of your vagina, but often most will stay hidden inside you.

The placenta is the link between you and your baby, providing essential energy, nutrients and oxygen. If that connection is disturbed in any way, it can seriously affect the health and wellbeing of your unborn child. If the abruption is big, it could potentially put your life and that of your baby at risk.

Signs and symptoms of placental abruption

A placental abruption is really painful. The bleeding can stimulate the womb to contract, so there will be labour-type pains. However, as well as the painful contractions there will also be pain that lasts in between contractions. This should not happen in normal labour.

Your womb will tighten up and can feel firm to the touch. Medical professionals describe it as 'woody hard' which may give you an indication of the feeling. You may notice some vaginal bleeding. This may be heavy or misleadingly light because as much as a third of the blood will stay inside you. The blood loss can make you feel extremely unwell, pale, weak and faint.

If the abruption has affected your baby, you may notice that their movements have decreased and they are less active.

Treatment of placental abruption

A placental abruption is an absolute emergency, so if you've got signs, get help straight away. It's not something that's safe to monitor at home or to wait patiently for a call back from your midwife or the labour ward. By acting quickly, you can help protect your health as well as the little life growing inside you.

The right treatment depends on how much of the placenta has come away from the womb, the wellbeing of you and your baby and how close to term you are. Sometimes it's safe to watch, monitor and see how things progress. If you are before term, your team may want to give you steroids to help your baby's lungs mature, so they have a better chance of breathing independently immediately after the birth.

Sometimes your obstetrician may decide to induce labour straight away. If it is thought that you or your baby could potentially be at risk, an emergency Caesarean will be done.

This must seem frightening, but the good news is that if treatment and delivery are swift, both you and your baby should make a rapid and straightforward recovery.

Placenta accreta

Placenta accreta is a rare condition where the placenta grows into the muscular wall of the uterus, usually at the site of a previous Caesarean scar. The placenta can invade the scar, growing into the wall of the womb. It makes it difficult to separate the placenta from the uterus and can lead to dangerous levels of bleeding.

Like an abruption, it sounds like a frightening condition. However, as a medical professional, I can assure you that we are all aware of the risks in women who have had previous sections. We are usually able to identify this condition on ultrasound and can find out more details with an MRI if necessary. Your medical team will work together to plan ahead so you can have a Caesarean section and a safe and healthy birth, although if the placenta cannot be removed, a hysterectomy may be advised. That is why careful planning of these deliveries is so important.

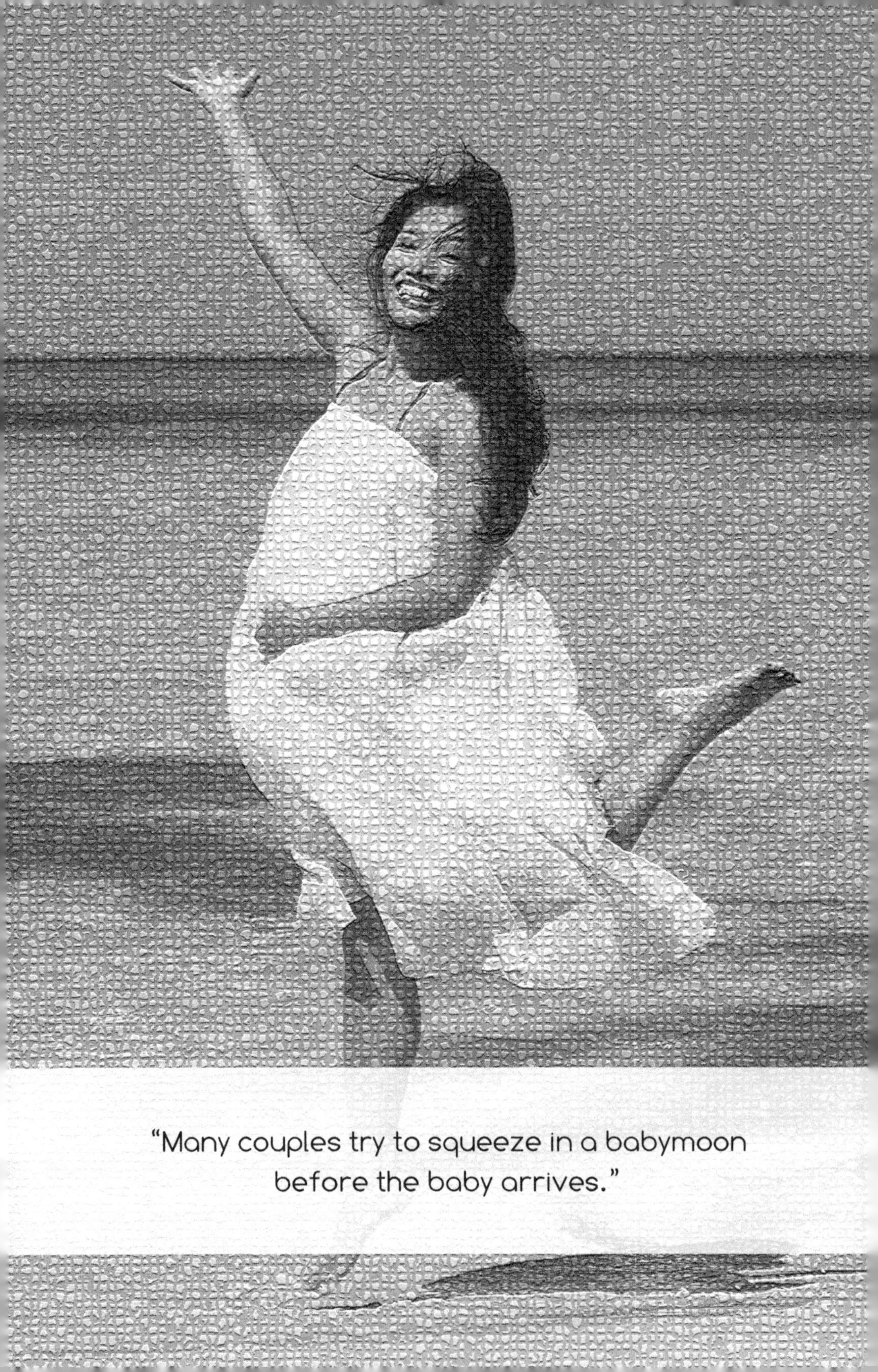

"Many couples try to squeeze in a babymoon before the baby arrives."

38

IS IT SAFE TO FLY IN PREGNANCY?

Whether you had already booked a holiday before finding out your happy news or are squeezing in a babymoon, pregnancy can be a great time to enjoy a last romantic break as a couple before the baby arrives. However, lots of women ask me this question because they are worried about flying in pregnancy, so what are the recommended rules?

The good news is, as long as your pregnancy is progressing well without any complications, flying shouldn't harm you or your baby. The evidence suggests that in a healthy pregnancy, any changes in air pressure or humidity shouldn't cause any problems or trigger miscarriage, pre-term labour or the early rupture of your waters. It is true that each and every person who flies is exposed to a very slight increase in radiation. However, this is not thought to be a risk if you only fly occasionally.

When should I fly?

Some women avoid travelling in the first trimester because they feel sick and tired. However, many people are already committed to holidays when they find out they're pregnant and continue with no problems. It's about choosing what's best for you and not overdoing things.

When it comes to air travel, the safest time to fly is now believed to be before 37 weeks. After this stage, you could theoretically go into labour at any moment, which could be a little challenging thousands of miles up in the air. If you're pregnant with twins, the increased risks of early labour mean that you can only fly before 32 weeks. But don't take our word for it. Check the rules with your airline and your travel insurer before booking flights.

The final months of pregnancy are exhausting and uncomfortable, even without adding travel into the mix. Sometime mid-pregnancy, between thirteen weeks and six months may be that perfect sweet spot for a trip away.

Problems and panics

The side-effects of pregnancy combined with the side-effects of flying can mean that you may find travelling a little more uncomfortable than usual. You may notice:

- Swelling of your feet and ankles due to fluid retention
- A stuffy nose and difficulty 'popping' your ears and equilibrating the pressure
- Sickness (motion during the flight can make pregnancy nausea worse)
- When you are pregnant you are at increased risk of developing a **DVT**. That risk increases when you fly, especially if it's long haul. A DVT or deep vein thrombosis is a blood clot that develops in the deep veins of your leg or pelvis. There is a danger of bits breaking off and travelling to your lungs (a condition known as a pulmonary embolism), which could put your life in danger

How can I help myself?

The good news is there's lots you can do to stay safe and comfortable as you take to the skies:

- Wear loose clothing and comfortable shoes.
- Wear your seatbelt below your bump, ask for an extension strap if it feels too tight.
- Sip plenty of water and pack healthy snacks to stave off hunger and nausea.
- Get up and walk around as much as you can and do stretches and ankle rotations in your seat.
- Reserve your seat in advance to guarantee extra legroom or an aisle seat.
- Longer flights of more than five hours can increase your risk of developing clots in the deep veins of your legs and pelvis (DVT). Protect yourself by drinking plenty of water, moving regularly and wearing compression stockings to prevent swelling and keep your blood moving.

When would I be told not to fly?

Sometimes a medical condition or complication could mean that flying could put you or baby at risk. You will be advised not to fly if you:

- Are at risk of early labour
- Have severe anaemia
- Have had recent episodes of significant vaginal bleeding
- Suffer from serious medical problems such as heart and lung disease, or have sickle cell anaemia and have recently had a crisis

> *I was worried about flying abroad in both pregnancies, so we chose to go on holiday in the UK. I didn't want to end up in a foreign hospital if any problems arose. I made sure I took my pregnancy notes with me in case I needed any care whilst away.*
>
> **~ Sam, Northfields**

Travelling while pregnant—how to stay safe

Wherever you decide to go, find out what the medical care options are and ensure that you have good insurance. Look at the small print and ensure that medical care during labour, premature birth and changing flights because of problems are properly covered.

If you're travelling within Europe, it's a good idea to take an EHIC card too. If you're British the rules may change with Brexit, but for the next couple of years, the right to discounted rates in twenty-eight countries still stands.

Take your handheld maternity notes too, so if you need medical help the doctors have the relevant information. But keep them close at hand, in your hand luggage. You don't want them getting lost if your luggage goes astray.

Choose your destination with care

If you're in control of the venue, choose wisely. If you live in the UK, British or European breaks are perfect for pregnancy. The travel times are shorter, so no uncomfortable lengthy flights. Try to stay close to good healthcare. Isolated lodges in the middle of nowhere with no good transport links may be romantic, but how will you get medical attention if you need it?

It's better to stay away from areas where you need vaccinations or disease prevention. Places where there is a risk of mosquito-borne diseases, like malaria, dengue fever or zika should be avoided if possible. If there's no option, see your doctor or a travel health expert before you leave. They can advise on protection, precautions and which vaccinations are safe during pregnancy.

Vaccinations

A number of vaccines aren't safe in pregnancy, particularly those that contain live bacteria or viruses. For specific advice, you should see your GP, midwife or a travel health expert.

Infection protection

If you are travelling to exotic or far-flung destinations take extra care. There has been loads in the news about the risks of the zika virus but that certainly isn't the only mosquito-carried infection that you need to be careful about; malaria, dengue fever and chikungunya can affect your health and your developing baby.

Protect yourself against bites by covering up, avoiding watery areas at dusk and using mosquito nets and wire-screens. Mosquitoes are repelled by some strong natural scents like citronella, peppermint and eucalyptus, so burn a candle or warm a little in a bowl.

The government says that insect repellents containing up to 50% DEET are effective and safe for pregnant women.

Sampling local food can be a holiday highlight, but try to avoid foods that could cause stomach upsets and travellers' diarrhoea. The risky foods include a lot of the usual suspects that feature in our foods to avoid in pregnancy section, like seafood. You should also take care to drink bottled water, avoid ice and be cautious with salads and raw veggies which may have been washed in tap water.

What should I take with me?

It's important to be prepared for any eventuality, don't forget to pack:

- Your hand-held pregnancy notes
- Any medication you need
- Insurance documents and an EHIC card for Europe
- A letter from your doctor or midwife confirming that you are healthy and well and detailing your due date if you're over 28 weeks

Remember to rest and have lots of fun, and let me wish you *bon voyage!*

39

HOW CAN I GET A GOOD NIGHT'S SLEEP?

Nearly everyone has difficulty sleeping towards the end of pregnancy—and that includes your partner! It takes hours to manoeuvre your bump into a comfortable position, then you need a wee, your legs start cramping and you lie awake worrying whether you're going to be a good enough parent.

It's rumoured to be Mother Nature's wonderful way of priming you for sleepless nights ahead, although in my opinion you'd probably be better prepared after stockpiling nine months of sleep. It's difficult not to get frustrated and uptight, which makes the situation worse. But don't toss, turn and torment yourself. These tips can hopefully help you get the rest you need.

> *In my first two pregnancies, I found the first three months the worst, especially with Polly when I used to regularly fall asleep in front of the telly. This time it was much worse towards the end. I was trying to look after both of the girls and I felt so big and cumbersome. It was also really difficult to get comfortable in bed. In the end, I had to move into the spare room because the mattress was softer.*
>
> **~ Min, Manchester**

Control cramps

Cramps are your legs' way of protesting about the extra work you're making them do. They can be a pain, literally and metaphorically, and can have you leaping out of bed with a level of agility you probably forgot you possessed:

- Take it easy, make sure give you relax and put your feet up.
- Tuck into lots of calcium rich foods like dairy produce and sardines. A milky drink at bedtime may soothe you to sleep and help prevent cramps.
- Before bed, stretch out your muscles; it can make a difference.
- When a killer cramp strikes, stretch it out. Pull your toe up towards your shin to extend the cramping muscles. If you're not agile enough to reach, ask your partner to lend a hand.
- Massage the muscle or pop a hot flannel on the area to release the muscle spasm.
- A lovely bath of magnesium salts will help you relax at the end of your day.

Have a catnap

I tried napping, but I felt worse afterwards, sluggish and heavy, like I'd been drugged. With a bit of trial and error I worked out that shorter naps were better for me, so I used to set my alarm for twenty minutes and I was good to go.

~ Elizabeth, Swansea

A siesta can boost your energy, reduce stress and make you feel better. But you need to keep them short and sweet. A twenty to thirty-minute snooze will recharge your batteries but shouldn't stop you dropping off at night.

Go caffeine-free

Caffeine is a stimulant that will prevent you from falling asleep. Cut down on coffee, tea, colas and energy drinks, especially in the evenings. Instead, choose decaffeinated alternatives, such as calming chamomile tea or a warm milky drink, to soothe you to sleep.

Be screen sensible

Tablets, mobiles and TVs can be too mentally stimulating at night, and backlit screens have been shown to inhibit sleep. Keep the bedroom for snoozing and sex. Try reading a little before bed if it helps you switch off, and leave the technology for other times.

Toilet training

Your growing uterus means there's less room for your bladder to expand, so frequent trips to the loo are vital. If pregnancy has made your ankles puffy, the extra fluid will be absorbed back into the bloodstream as soon as you put your legs up in bed, making you need a wee in the middle of the night. It can be tricky to fall back to sleep, so help yourself:

- Make sure your bladder is totally empty before you go to bed by leaning forward while you wee so it empties properly.
- Decrease ankle swelling by putting your feet up in the evenings to allow the fluid to drain away.
- Have a final wee immediately before going to bed.

Too darn hot

Your baby is your own central heating system, boosting your metabolism and making you more sensitive to warm temperatures. Make sure your bedroom isn't too hot by opening a window at night and switching to a summer weight duvet if you're still overheating.

Stressbusting

You're about to be a parent as well as facing the challenges of birth, so a little excitement or anxiety is natural. Stress can keep you awake at night, so try to switch off with relaxation techniques like deep abdominal breathing, by using a self-hypnosis app or practising the relaxation exercises you've been taught at your antenatal classes.

Indigestion

There's only so much room in your abdomen and pelvis. Your growing womb pushes everything out of the way in the last trimester and leaves your stomach squashed. That, together with the hormones softening the stomach valves, can make the acidic stomach contents flow up into the gullet and give you burning pain and indigestion.

- Don't eat late at night.
- Prop the end of your mattress up with a few books so your head is higher than your tummy. It's a matter of gravity and makes it more difficult for the acid to flow back up the oesophagus.
- Settle your stomach at bedtime with a glass of milk, or ask your doctor or midwife for an antacid such as Gaviscon.

A relaxing bath

I mentioned my wife Sharon's top tip for insomnia back in the section on tiredness in the first trimester. Well, now's the time to restock your supplies of lavender and Epsom salts. A bath just before bedtime, with some Epsom salts and a splash of lavender oil will relax your muscles and help you unwind.

Get comfy

It's tricky to get comfy when you're heavily pregnant. Extra cushions can help provide support and comfort. Try popping a pillow between your knees and use another two to support your bump and back. Hopefully, there'll still be enough room for your partner!

The magic of massage

Encourage your partner to give you a massage at bedtime. As well as soothing your aching muscles, it provides an opportunity to spend time focusing on your relationship, not just the imminent arrival.

Mum's conundrum

I love to sleep on my tummy, will I squash my baby?

~ Liz, Leeds

Dr Keith says:

The good news is there's lots of fluid and a big muscly womb to protect your baby from any damage. However, as you get bigger you may struggle to get comfy on your tummy. You'll wobble around like a weeble on your bump! It's still safe to sleep face down, but you may find that turning your body a little to the side, supporting your bump with cushions, or even investing in a doughnut-shaped pillow can keep you a bit more comfortable.

Mum's conundrum

I've been sleeping on my back in pregnancy and it's making me snore. My boyfriend keeps complaining. How can I stop?

~ Ali, Bristol

Dr Keith says:

I'm sorry, but I'm on your boyfriend's side here—but not because of the snoring, that's common in pregnancy because the hormones make the lining of your nose swell. It's because after the first trimester it's really not a good idea to lie flat on your back. The womb can press down on the vena cava, which is the big vein that sends blood back to the heart. The blood supply can fall, leaving you weak, dizzy and short of breath and affecting the blood supply to your baby too. Try lying on your side instead. It'll be better for your baby—and your boyfriend!

40

WHAT ARE THE PREGNANCY SYMPTOMS I SHOULDN'T IGNORE?

Sometimes there are so many body changes and challenges in pregnancy, that it can be difficult to tell what's normal and what's definitely not. Often, mums don't want to bother their doctor and will sit on symptoms that could indicate something serious. So here's my don't-hang-around-get-on the-phone list.

Many of these symptoms and conditions are covered in more detail elsewhere in this book. However, I wanted to put them in one place so anyone reading knows at a glance what to do.

If your symptoms are severe or your baby isn't moving, get in contact with the labour ward urgently. Trust your instincts—even if there turns out to be nothing wrong, it's better to be safe than sorry.

Call your pregnancy doctor checklist

- **Vaginal bleeding**
  Bleeding in pregnancy can be worrying. Often it's harmless spotting, or closer to term it could be an exciting indication that your baby may be on their way. However, it could indicate problems like a bleed behind the placenta, especially if you've got pain, so it is important to get in touch with your healthcare team.

In my first pregnancy, I had some bleeding in my fifth and sixth week so I went to A&E and was referred to the early pregnancy unit to be given a scan to see if everything was OK. I also had reduced movements in my first pregnancy which I got checked out to be told all was fine. It's better to get a check-up if you're worried.

~ Sam, Northfields

- **High fever**
  It's normal to get hot and bothered in pregnancy. Your baby is your internal furnace, boosting your metabolism and making you more sensitive to warm temperatures. But that shouldn't make you feel feverish, shivery or unwell.

  If your temperature is raised, you may be suffering from an infection. That could be something relatively harmless like a cold, but it could also indicate a disease that could endanger you or your baby. Raised temperatures during pregnancy could suggest a urinary tract infection or a virus that can affect your unborn child, like toxoplasmosis.

  If your temperature is more than 37.5 degrees centigrade, consider arranging a check-up, but if it's more than 39 degrees centigrade, it is more likely to be due to a significant infection, so get medical help immediately.

- **Severe itching, especially of the hands or feet**
  A little itchiness is normal in pregnancy, but if it's severe, especially if it's associated with jaundice, it could indicate the rare but serious complication, cholestasis.

  Obstetric cholestasis can pose a significant risk to the health of your developing baby and can even lead to stillbirth, so it's essential to get medical advice if you spot the symptoms.

It happened to me

I was having a relatively easy pregnancy with my second child when I started to get itchy feet and hands, especially at night, at around 36 weeks. I went to my GP but I really didn't feel too concerned and the doctor seemed relatively relaxed too. She took blood to send to be checked. I left the GP's room having been reassured that I wouldn't hear anything unless there was a problem.

I continued to itch and slept intermittently by putting cold flannels on my intensely itchy feet. I didn't hear anything for a week when I was rung up by the hospital. The results showed that I had obstetric cholestasis and they recommended that I should have an early delivery—that day. With the midwife's help, my husband and I chose to give our baby a chance to come by himself. They agreed that we could try inducing the baby with a sweep. Forty-eight hours later, despite some mild contractions, there was no real progress and so they broke my waters first thing with a plan to move on to induction drugs if necessary later in the day. After a stomp around the hospital grounds and a little lunch, my son was born at 12.30 pm. I was grateful that I was given the chance to have as natural a birth as possible despite the OC.

~ Lara, West Sussex

- **Decreased baby movement**
  Get help immediately if you're worried about your baby's movements. An active baby is a healthy baby, and if your baby may be becoming distressed, time is of the essence. I've said this before, but it bears repeating: don't wait and sleep on it, speak to your midwife, doctor or the labour ward straight away, no matter what time of day or night it is.

- **Sickness that stops you keeping fluids down**
  It's essential not to ignore recurrent vomiting such that you are unable to keep anything down. This severe form of pregnancy sickness is known as **hyperemesis gravidarum**. It is a serious but rare condition. If you are unable to keep fluids down or are not passing urine frequently ,see your doctor who will check your urine for ketones. You may need to go into hospital for anti-sickness medication and re-hydration by a drip.

- **Leak of fluid from the vagina**
  If you notice a gush or trickle of fluid from your vagina, your waters may have broken. Amniotic fluid is clear and a pale straw-like colour, so it can look an awful lot like urine, but it smells different and you'll have no control over the flow.

  The management will depend on your stage of pregnancy, but at any time, if you think your waters have broken early, you should be assessed at the hospital. If it is early, a swab will be taken to exclude infection and you may have a scan to assess how much fluid is left around your baby. If your waters have definitely broken, you'll usually be admitted and monitored for a couple of days to check your baby is well and that there's no fever or other sign of infection.

- **Pain passing water, especially if you are also feeling feverish and unwell**
  Burning or stabbing pain when you pass water, particularly if the urine is a little smelly or blood-tinged, could indicate a urine infection. These can be more serious in pregnancy, with an increased risk of spread to the kidneys and the blood and the danger of triggering early labour, so it's important to get medical help.

- **Severe and persistent headache**
  Headaches are common, whether you're pregnant or not. Dehydration, stress, migraines and caffeine withdrawal can trigger pain. However, severe head pain can be caused by pre-eclampsia, which affects ten per cent of pregnancies.

  Women with this condition may feel perfectly well at first, although it may be associated with sudden swelling, abdominal pain, visual disturbances and headache.

  If left untreated, pre-eclampsia may put both you and your baby at risk, so if you're worried, get checked straight away.

- **Sudden and widespread swelling**
  Puffiness in pregnancy is to be expected, but sudden and severe swelling (especially if it's widespread and affecting the face) could be a sign of pre-eclampsia.

- **Visual disturbance such as blurring or spots before the eyes**
  Blurry vision and other problems with your eyesight can be another indication that you may be developing pre-eclampsia.

- **Sudden sharp tummy pain**
  As well as the more common symptoms of pre-eclampsia, like headache and swelling, some women may notice severe

sharp pain below the ribs on the right. This can be caused by a serious, but thankfully uncommon, form of pre-eclampsia called HELLP syndrome. It affects the liver and the blood's ability to clot effectively, and all women affected need urgent medical attention.

- **Severe thirst together with fatigue and passing more urine**
  Lots of pregnant women need to go to the loo frequently and tiredness is a common symptom too—but together with thirst, recurrent infections and blurred vision, these symptoms could suggest you may be developing gestational diabetes.

- **Sudden or increasing pelvic pain**
  Aching pain on movement is common with pelvic girdle problems in pregnancy. However, sudden and severe pain in the womb could indicate a placental abruption. This is a serious condition in which the placenta partially or completely separates from your womb which could deprive your baby of oxygen and nutrients, and cause severe bleeding that can be dangerous to you both. Signs of a placental abruption include vaginal bleeding, but sometimes the blood stays in the uterus behind the placenta, so you might not see any bleeding at all.

- **Painful abdominal cramps and contractions**
  In the last few months of pregnancy, abdominal pain is usually an indication that your womb is getting fit and flexed for birth. The main concern at this time is that you may be going into labour too soon.

  If you're feeling regular, painful cramps that are building in intensity, call your doctor, midwife or the delivery suite immediately. This is especially important if you have noticed a little blood, a mucous show or some fluid leaking. Once you're past 37 weeks, it's time to get your bag and call your birth partner—your baby could be on their way. The contact numbers for your doctor, your midwife and the labour ward will be in the front of your antenatal notes.

Dr Keith says:

Never be worried about getting help if you're not sure everything is OK. If in doubt, go to hospital. It's better to be safe than sorry!

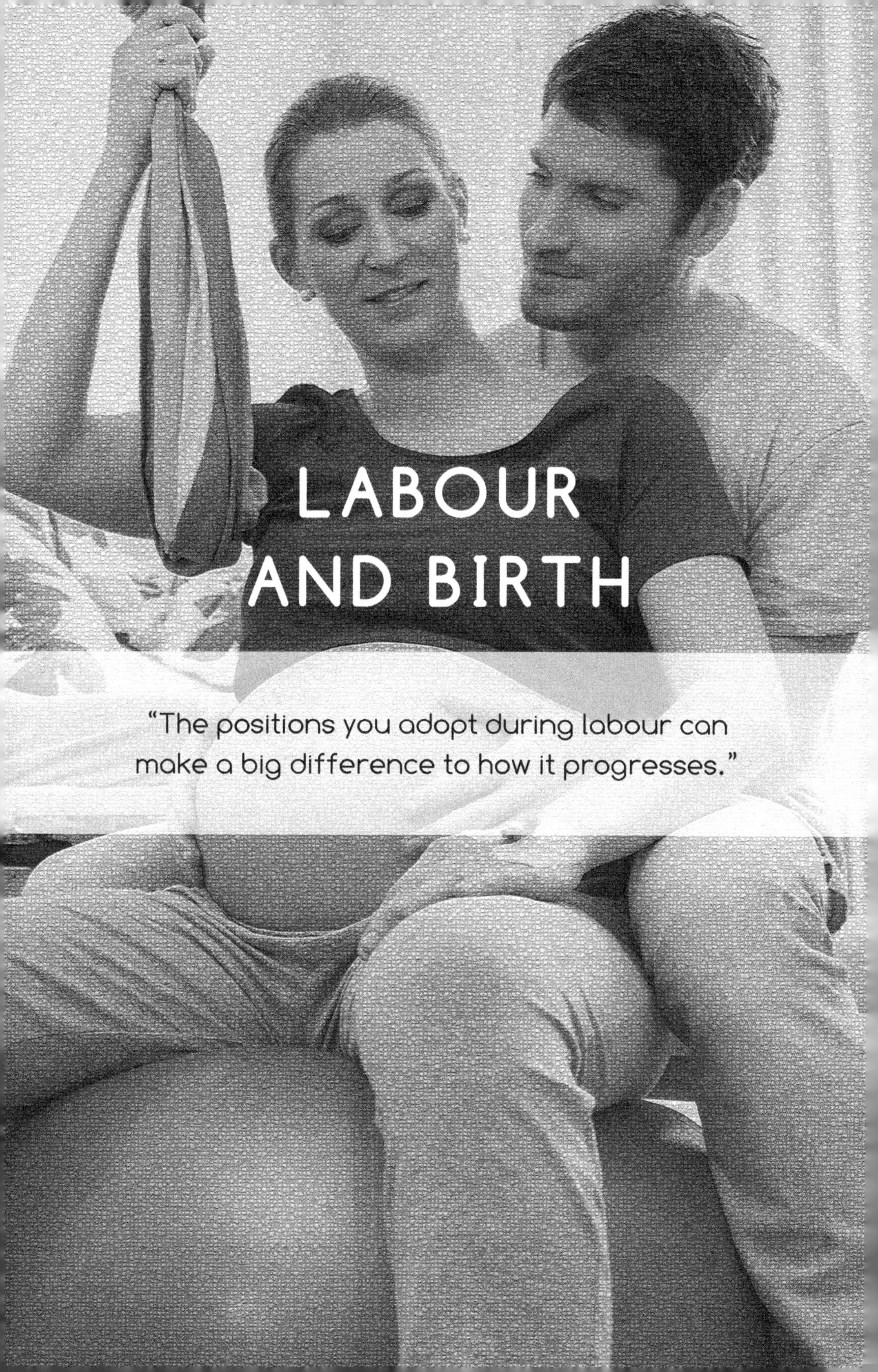

LABOUR AND BIRTH

"The positions you adopt during labour can make a big difference to how it progresses."

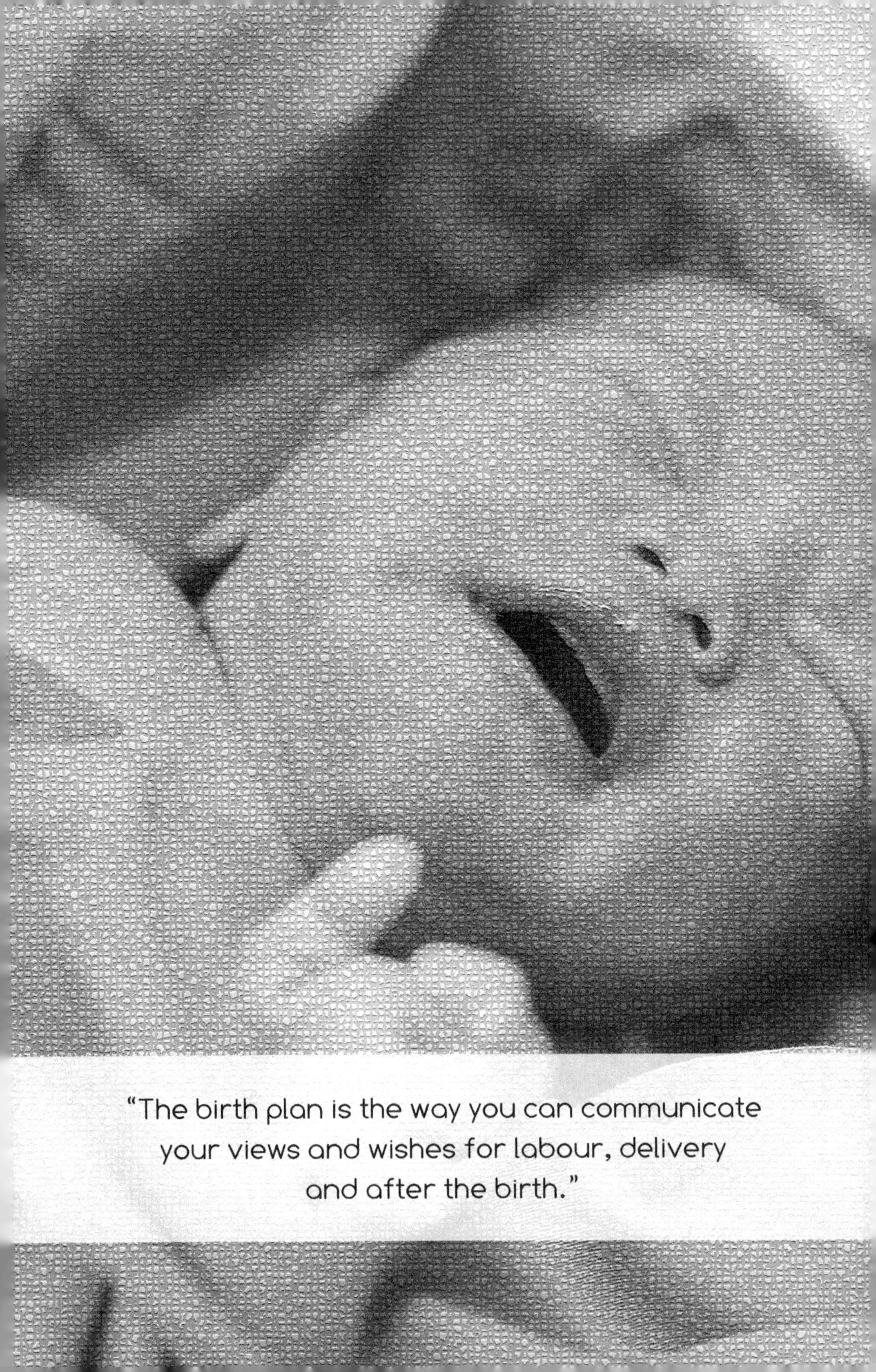

"The birth plan is the way you can communicate your views and wishes for labour, delivery and after the birth."

41

HOW CAN I GET READY FOR THE BIRTH?

Hospitals can be intimidating and scary, so planning to deliver your baby can be a time of stress as well as anticipation. As you start counting down to 40 weeks, your body and your baby will naturally begin to get themselves ready for the big day. You can get your head around the idea too by giving some thought to what lies ahead.

Each and every birth is different, so it's impossible to make fixed plans—but with some thought, preparation and organisation, you can make life and labour that little bit easier.

> *My preparation was not to think about it too early! There was a big baby in there. It's coming out one way or another and there is no point in over thinking or stressing out about it. At the end of the day, labour is only a day of pain—you can cope with anything for one day!*
>
> **~ Lindsey, Kilkeel**

Antenatal classes

Antenatal or parent-craft classes can be a fantastic source of knowledge and support. As well as helping you learn about the intricacies of labour, they'll also get you ready and confident for the birth. Many mums tell me that the classes are a waste of time because they can get the information they need online. I don't agree. They're a real opportunity to meet new people, share your experiences and exchange tips. Many of the women I know and have cared for have made friends for life at their antenatal groups.

What classes?

Your doctor and midwife will have information about local classes and any independent groups. You could also check-out NCT classes near to you. Places get booked up really quickly, so ask early in pregnancy to not miss out. You're free to attend more than one series of classes. NHS-led midwife classes are usually free, but there will be a charge for NCT sessions.

Some classes are exclusively for pregnant women, while others welcome dads and partners to some or all of the sessions. If you're a single mother, a teenage mum, you're expecting a multiple birth or if English is not your first language ask your midwife or health centre if there are any special classes that could suit you. In some areas, different groups are run, but that absolutely doesn't mean you are excluded from the general classes if you'd prefer to attend those.

Staying local is sensible. You'll learn about the specific options for labour and birth in your area and it'll be easy to be meet up with group members for a coffee and a chat after your babies arrive.

What happens?

All classes differ, but I can assure you that you won't be sitting in rows behind desks. It's definitely not like going back to school. The sessions are friendly, relaxed and fun. It's a two-way process, with people asking questions, talking about their own experiences and sharing a laugh together.

Most classes start between 8 and 10 weeks before your baby is due, so around the time when you are 30 to 32 weeks pregnant, although you should start a little earlier, at 24 weeks, if you're expecting twins or more. They're held once a week and last a couple of hours. You can usually choose a daytime or evening session, depending on what works best for you.

What will I learn?

The classes will cover all sorts of topics from your diet, fitness and health in pregnancy to what happens during labour and birth, including information about pain relief and how to cope in labour.

You may have seen films where the whole group practises relaxation and breathing techniques and I'm glad to say that for many groups, that image is still a reality. You may feel awkward and embarrassed at first, but it's a great way to bond as a group, good preparation for the big day and something to laugh about later.

The midwife or group leader will tell you about different kinds of birth, including instrumental deliveries such as ventouse or forceps and Caesarean sections. All the information can help you form and fine-tune your birth plan.

Later classes may talk about your health after the birth, your feelings, breastfeeding and the highs and lows of caring for your baby.

What can I do if I can't make classes?

You don't need classes to have a good birth experience or to be a great mum. If you simply can't get there, speak to your healthcare team. They'll give you lots of information, tell you how to arrange a tour of your hospital or birthing centre and may even have DVDs about antenatal care. On YourPregnancyDoctor.com you can sign up for video courses available for each stage of pregnancy, from the first missed period to those early days with your new baby.

Mums' opinions

For me antenatal classes were not useful, they were far too long and too much for me as I was working full time. I found it a burden to sit in a class for two hours whilst heavily pregnant. I found online tools much more informative.

~ Kirsty, Annalong

I wasn't offered any classes and didn't know how you could arrange them. This makes me feel like I missed out, as some friends have since done NCT courses and met lifelong friends, I wish I'd had more information on this, as it's something I would like to have done, but I didn't know it was available.

~ Sam, Northfields

I loved antenatal classes, I learned so much and I made a group of friends that have stayed together. My babies are adults now—but I still meet up with the women I met at that time.

~ Philippa , Gloucester

Your birth plan

The birth plan is your way of communicating your feelings and wishes for labour to your midwife or doctor. It should cover everything from pain relief to positions, partners and feeding preferences. You can find out more about the questions to consider later in this section. However, as I recommend to all the women I care for, try to introduce some flexibility into your plan—and into your mind. A birth plan can provide a great template, but many women change their minds once they're in labour. Alternatively, there may be complications and your baby may have a birth plan of their own. So it's important not to be too fixed in your thinking.

The early bird...

There's an old army saying that prior planning and preparation prevents p*** poor performance. They're right. Although a military campaign is probably unnecessary, it's a good idea to get your stuff together for labour and birth before you have to pant your way through contractions.

Pack your bags by the time you reach 36 weeks, so there are no last-minute panics if your little one decides to make an early break for the outside world. You can find checklists and everything you need to know in the next section. Maybe think about having three separate bags. One for labour, one for you and your baby after the birth and another stuffed with snacks, entertainment, contact numbers and of course a phone and a camera for your birth partner.

Fill the freezer

The days and weeks after the birth can pass in a blur. Sleepless nights, endless nappy changes, establishing feeding and recovering from the birth can mean that there's simply no time or energy to cook or go shopping. Plan ahead and fill the fridge, freezer and store cupboard with nutritious and easy to prepare snacks and meals.

It can be a good idea to set up some online shops in advance too. You'll stay topped up with fresh produce and you'll never be caught short of loo roll, toiletries, nappies and sanitary towels.

Sort the paperwork

You're unlikely to remember to pay the gas bill if it's due the day after the birth. So get ahead and set up payment in advance. Or consider organising to pay by direct debit and you may save a few quid too.

Know the numbers

Keep a list of essential numbers close at hand for when you go into labour. Don't rely on programming them into your mobile, because sod's law says that you'll run out of charge at the vital moment. You'll need the number of the labour ward, your partner's phone number, your hospital reference number and a taxi contact in case of emergencies.

Your chariot awaits

How are you planning to get to the hospital? Know the route, how long it takes and any sneaky rat runs or shortcuts. Don't let your car run low on petrol; if you're stuck waiting for emergency services there's no guarantee that your baby will be as patient. Buy a car seat and make sure you know how to fit it, so you can whisk your new baby home in comfort and safety.

> *I thought I was ready for the birth but nothing could have prepared me for the reality. The way to the hospital was a familiar route. However, part of the road was closed. We nearly panicked—but my husband drove through the roadblock! Haha! I didn't have a specific birth plan, just that I wasn't opposed to pain relief when I needed it.*
>
> **~ Kirsty, Annalong**

Getting big sister or brother on board

A new family member brings enormous changes and that can be difficult for older children to take. Pregnancy is a time of excitement and upheaval, and everything is often focused on planning and preparing for the new arrival.

Appointments, scans and tests can occupy Mum and Dad's time during the pregnancy, which can make existing children feel understandably unsettled and uncertain. When your new little one arrives, it won't get any easier. Let's be honest, newborn babies consume a huge amount of energy and attention. It's common for older siblings to feel excluded and jealous of the baby, which they may demonstrate by either becoming silent and withdrawn or acting out.

The good news is that there's loads you can do to prepare your kids for their new baby brother or sister. By being sensitive, planning ahead and responding to their needs you can continue to have a happy family, with each member feeling important and valued.

It worked for me:

We kept talking about the new baby all the time! Joshua is three and so time doesn't mean a lot to him, so to tell him the baby was coming when I was three months pregnant was no different than telling him at nine months!

We had a present bought for his first meeting with the baby. We also made sure he was the first to meet the new baby and that he got to show the new baby off to other visitors. Plenty of cuddles reassured him that he was still Mummy's boy! Joshua pure loves his wee brother and I think good preparation had a lot to do with that.

~ Lindsey, Kilkeel

We used to encourage our older daughter to come to some appointments where she could listen to her heart beat. She would talk to her little sister when we sat on the couch together. We also bought presents for them to give to each other when the baby was born, something special from their sister.

~ Sam, Northfields

- **Make an early start**
  Let your little one know that a baby is on the way. Try to explain in terms they understand. Offer them relatable frames of reference; maybe a friend at nursery or a cousin has had a baby sister. Kids can be impatient and may expect a baby to appear in five minutes, or tomorrow at the absolute latest. Let them know in ways they can comprehend. Just before their birthday when it's warm and sunny, after Christmas or one hundred sleeps to go.

- **Let your child be your guide**
  Children are inquisitive and will ask the questions that they want answered. Where is it? Where did it come from? Don't feel you need to give long complex and scientific explanations; be honest but age appropriate. A simple short answer is probably all they want. Depending on their age and understanding explaining 'it's in Mummy's tummy' and 'Daddy put a seed in there' may be enough. If they want to know more, I can assure you they'll keep questioning. Reading a book together can help if you're struggling to find the right words.

- **Show them the way**
  Too much talking may bore your little one. Instead, try helping them picture what's going to happen by visiting friends with babies, looking through their infant photos, or taking

them to an appointment so they can hear the heartbeat and sharing ideas for baby names.

If they're interested in babies and caring, buying or borrowing a baby doll, pram or car-seat may grab their attention. You can show them how you look after and care for a new baby. They can even get a little nappy changing practice in!

- **Planning for childbirth**

  Make plans for childbirth well in advance. Who will look after them? Will they stay at home or with a relative? Make sure your little one understands exactly what is going to happen, so they are not shocked and upset on the day. For many children, a day with Grandma and Grandpa or a close family friend can be a treat to look forward to.

- **After the birth**

  It's a good idea to consider letting your child visit you and the new baby in hospital as soon as possible after the birth. It's better if they come alone, without grandparents or anyone else taking over and monopolising the baby and the conversation. A lovely quiet time can help them meet their new baby brother or sister and start to recognise that you are still a close, intimate family unit, just a bit of a bigger one.

  Understand that it can be tough on your older child when the new baby is showered with pressies. Sometimes it can help if you prepare a special gift the baby has brought them to say thank you for being their big brother or sister.

- **Bringing baby home**

  When you bring the baby home, try to make sure you also maintain your other children's routines. That means continuing with nursery, school or toddler groups. It can seem harsh to send them away—but maintaining the regular rhythms of day will really help them adapt.

Include them in the daily care of the baby so they feel involved, not excluded. You may find that you have a willing helper to hand. Be sensitive and patient, even if it means that every task may take twice as long. Running and fetching nappies, cuddling and burping baby or gently rocking their chair can make them feel important and useful.

If your child is not interested in the baby, don't panic, that's normal too. Don't force things. Instead, keep engaging with them and involving them. They'll come around in time.

Breastfeeding can be particularly tough. Your hands and your body are busy; your child is excluded and they may target this time to try to gain attention and get you to do something important to them. Plan your distraction techniques, have toys to hand, read them a story or rely on a favourite TV programme to keep them happy and occupied.

- **One-on-one**
  Make sure you still spend special time with them every day. It's important to have time together when you aren't occupied by the new arrival. When baby is asleep, or your partner is on duty, give your older child undivided attention. You'll both benefit from the closeness and your older child will be reassured that they're still your baby too.

And finally, some wise words from a mother I cared for:

I think every pregnancy guide should have a mini section on being prepared for the baby. I think so many women have focused on the pregnancy and birth and are underprepared for what comes after! Even if it is a reminder to read a couple of baby books and to get some helplines under your belt!

Yes, you get the baby clothes and the cot and the buggy—but what the hell do you do with the tiny thing that is suddenly so precious and your responsibility? I was not too badly prepared, but I still looked at this tiny being and wondered what now? Luckily, the midwife stayed with us for a bath, dressing and bed! In previous generations, you lived with your family and everyone rallied around and top tips were passed generation to generation. I'm not sure this exists so much today.

~ Amy, London

Although this book finishes with the delivery, you'll find more information to prepare you for birth and beyond on YourPregnancy Doctor.com.

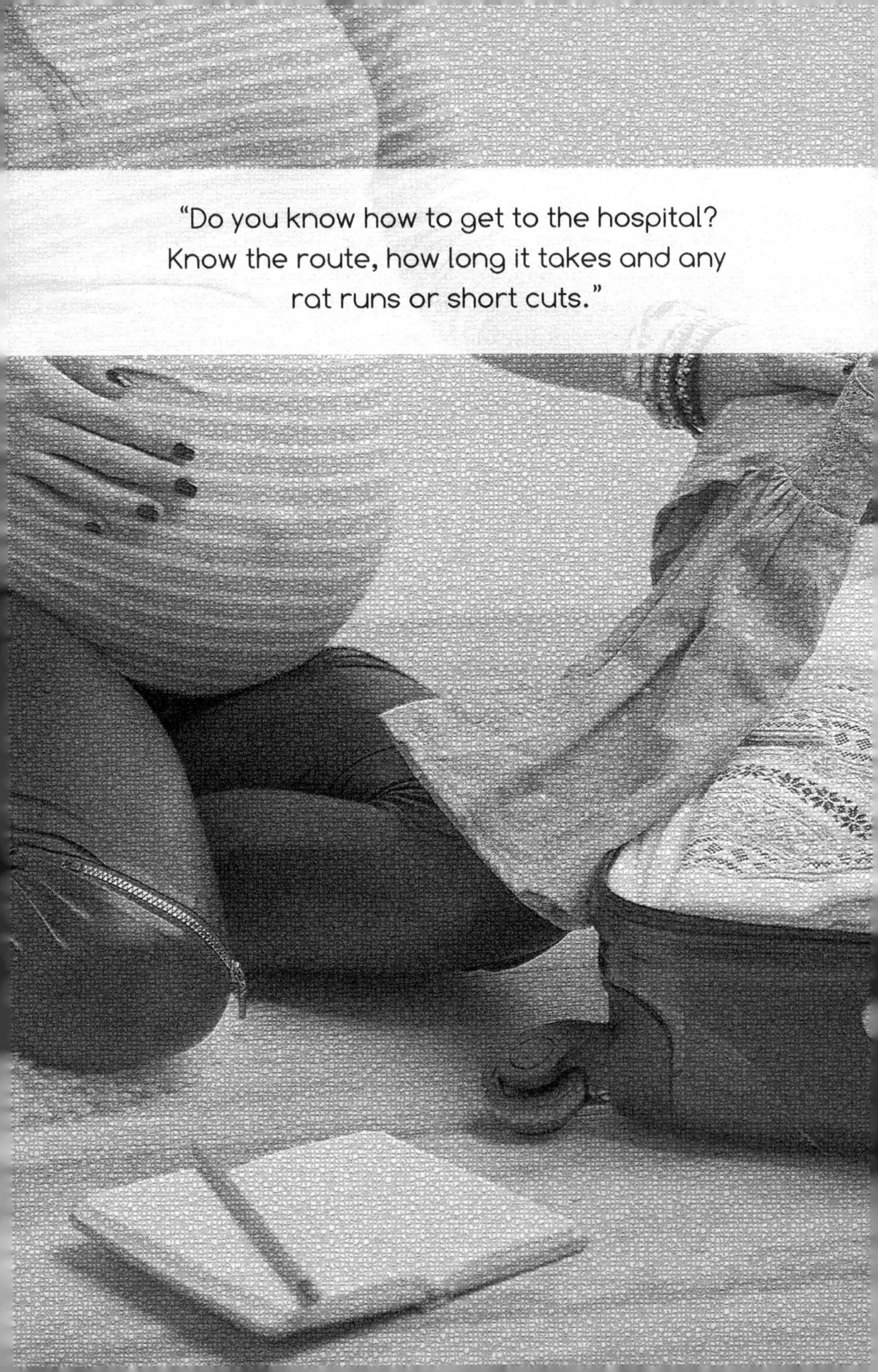

"Do you know how to get to the hospital? Know the route, how long it takes and any rat runs or short cuts."

42

WHAT SHOULD I PACK IN MY HOSPITAL BAG?

It's so exciting packing your bag for the big day. Suddenly, everything feels real. It's a good idea to be prepared before you reach 36 weeks, in case your little one decides to make an early debut. There's a lot to think about, but armed with my check-lists you should have all you need for the birth and for your amazing new baby.

All you need for labour

- Maternity notes and your birth plan
- Nightshirt or other comfy sleepwear
- Dressing gown
- Socks and slippers
- Towel and flannel or sponge, to stay fresh (a facial water mist can be cooling and refreshing, too)
- Hairband or bobbles to keep your hair out of your face
- Books, magazines or downloaded films to keep you occupied during quiet moments
- Phone, charger, back-up battery pack and headphones
- Lip salve or vaseline for dry lips

- Massage oil with essential oils if you want to use aromatherapy
- Water and snacks to stay hydrated and sustain your energy

All you need for your baby

- Three vests
- Threes sleepsuits
- Nappies
- Wipes
- Nappy cream
- Socks, booties and scratch mittens
- Cotton wool
- Baby blanket for swaddling
- Going home outfit with coat or shawl for the first outing in the big wide world

All you need for after the birth

- Your washbag and toiletries
- Disposable pants and maternity pads, not glamorous but oh so useful
- Two nursing bras and breast pads
- Button fronted nightwear for easy breastfeeding access
- Mobile phone, charger and spare battery pack
- Hairbrush and makeup
- Change and cash for food or vending machines
- Comfortable clothes and shoes for travelling home (don't be too ambitious; you won't be squeezing into your old jeans yet)

All your partner needs

- A copy of your birth plan
- Contact list for passing on the good news

- Phone, charger and back-up battery pack
- Camera, if they don't use their phone
- Change of t-shirt, in case they get a little messy too
- Books, magazine or downloaded films
- Snacks and drinks
- Cash and change for food, vending machines and parking charges

Mums' tips

I forgot a towel when I had my first and it was difficult to get one, so definitely put one in the bag. Talc is also good because hospitals are so warm—it was good to stop you sweating.

~ Lindsey, Kilkeel

My big recommendation is packing paper knickers. The blood floods through everything and who wants to spend time washing grubby underwear? The disposable ones were big and comfy and less hassle all round.

~ Philippa, Gloucester

I think you should pack something warm. I got shivery after the birth and would have loved to have had a fleecy blanket or shawl or something. Instead, I had to use a hospital towel and scratchy blanket. Next time I'm going to definitely pack something soft and snuggly for me, not just the baby.

~ Fi, Leeds

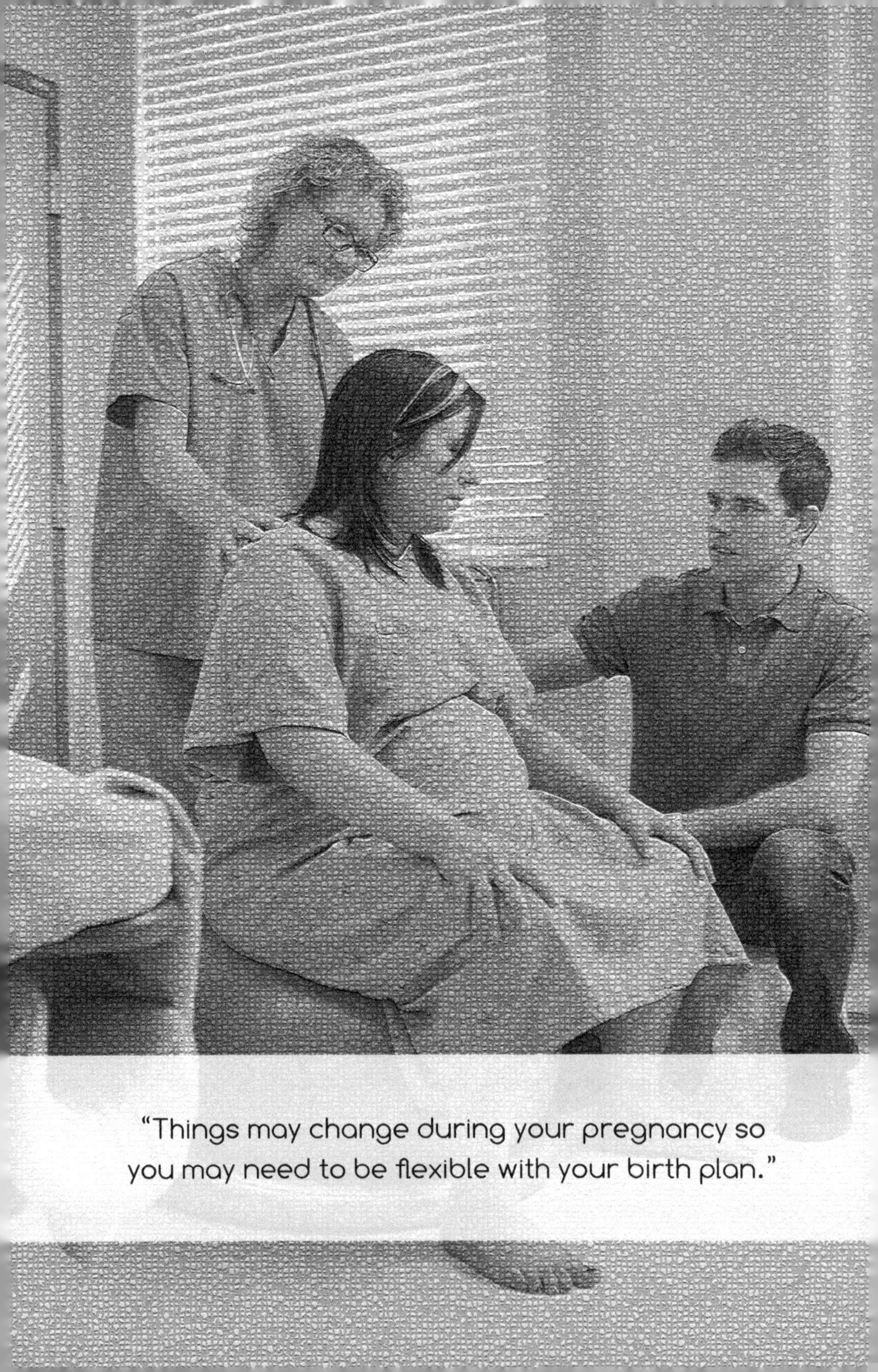
"Things may change during your pregnancy so you may need to be flexible with your birth plan."

43

WHAT SHOULD I PUT IN MY BIRTH PLAN?

A birth plan is your way of expressing your preferences and priorities for the sort of birth you would like. By writing down what you want to happen, and what you'd ideally hope to avoid, you can communicate your thoughts and wishes to the healthcare professional who is going to care for you and help you deliver your baby.

Why do I need a plan?

Like most pregnancy healthcare professionals, I ask expectant mums to produce a birth plan. Not because I don't know what to do, or because I will ever do anything other than what is best for mum and baby, it's simply because I want to actively involve the mother in the decision-making process.

A plan isn't compulsory, so you can go with the flow if you prefer—but if you have specific views about what you want, or don't want, during labour, it really helps if the people looking after you know what these things are.

What is it all about?

When it comes to birth, there's an awful lot to consider. Your obstetrician, doctor or midwife should help you prepare and perfect your plan. I'll go into more detail later in this section-but here's a handy checklist, to help you cover the most important questions.

Birth plan checklist

- Who do I want as my birth partner?
- Where do I want to deliver my baby?
- How do I want to deliver my baby?
- What pain relief would I prefer?
- Do I want my baby delivered straight onto my body or cleaned and wrapped first?
- If my labour doesn't progress, what intervention would I prefer?
- Am I happy for drugs to be used to speed up my labour?
- What would I prefer if my labour has to be induced?
- What are my feelings about instrumental deliveries?
- What are my feelings about Caesarean sections?
- What do I think about episiotomies?
- Do I want an injection to be given to speed up the delivery of the placenta in the third stage?
- Do I want my baby to be given an injection of vitamin K after the birth to prevent bleeding problems?
- How am I planning to feed my baby?

I'm now going to emphasise something I say to every mother I care for: it's important to remember that a birth plan is a guide and not a guarantee. What everyone wants most is a healthy baby and a healthy mum. If something happens to threaten either you or your baby, plans will have to be changed. I think it is helpful to think of this as revising your birth plan, even if you have to do it quickly.

> *I did have a loose birth plan, but it was the opposite of what happened. I was keen for a vaginal birth and not a Caesarean but was happy to have interventions if necessary for the safety of the baby.*
>
> **~ Andrea, London**

You need to trust the doctor or midwife who is going to attend your delivery. If circumstances change, you need to understand they're doing the right thing. It's also important to have a partner with you, whom you trust completely and who can understand what's going on when you may be in pain and under stress. That person has to be prepared to help change the birth plan in your place, if necessary.

> *We discussed our wishes for the birth with our midwife in advance. I wanted a calm natural birth with as few drugs as possible and prepared for birth using a hypnobirthing CD. In the end, I ended up being induced five days before the due date due to poor fetal growth.*
>
> **~ Laurie, London**

Researching your birth plan

When you're putting together your birth plan, it's important to find out as much about your birth options as possible. By gathering information from a variety of different sources, you can start to compose a picture of the sort of birth you would like to experience.

Ask the experts

Your obstetrician, GP or midwife will offer plenty of their extensive knowledge and advice. They may give you leaflets and recommend trusted information sources. I know that antenatal appointments can sometimes be hectic and a little overwhelming, so if you have specific questions, it can help to write them down so your mind doesn't go blank at the critical moment.

Get out and about

It's a good idea to visit the hospital, clinic or birthing centre in which you're considering giving birth. Most offer group tours, or you could ask if you and your partner can have a proper look around on your own. It can help you get a feel for the environment and ethos, so you can see if it seems like the right place for your baby to be born.

Net knowledge

There's a huge amount of information available online, some is fantastic and some is frankly dangerous and it can be difficult to tell the safe from the suspect. That's the reason I started **Your Pregnancy Doctor**, so you can be sure that the information you access is accurate and considers the safety of you and your baby above everything else.

Been there, done that

Personal experiences and recommendations can be incredibly useful, and can really help you picture and understand the whole incredible process of childbirth. Chat to friends and family members who have been through birth or have played an active role in supporting a partner. They can tell you about the pros and cons of the choices they made—from pain-relief, to the good and bad bits about birth in your local hospital unit and birthing centre, to the right obstetrician to oversee your care. Many of the women I care for have come to me after a recommendation from a friend whose baby I delivered.

Lessons and learning

Sign up for antenatal classes. They're a great opportunity to meet new people, exchange tips and learn about the nitty-gritty of labour. Classes may be run out of your local health centre. Alternatively, talk to your obstetrician, GP or midwife about any independent groups running in your area.

My 'plan' was to have as natural a birth as possible. I like 'plans', I like to feel in control. After researching other people's birthing stories and discussing the topic openly with family and friends I felt prepared. I had booked the birthing pool at the hospital and was determined that everything would go as envisaged. I was that expectant mother with her hospital bag prepared by my front door weeks before my due date.

I woke on the 14th April at my usual time of approximately 8am. I felt terrible pains and at 37 weeks I excitedly rang my sister who, along with my husband, was to be my birthing partner. Once at the hospital I was pleased that I had involved her as she proved to be a fantastic support.

I soon regretted that I had opted against the pain relief offered. By the time I realised I wanted to suppress the pain, which had become almost unbearable, it was too late. I was offered the water birth pool but I couldn't imagine anything worse; I wanted my baby out!

~ Hayley, Blackpool

Team talk

You, your birth partner and the practitioner who will deliver your baby are a team, so chat to your partner about the type of labour and birth you would like, how they envisage their role and any worries they may have.

As you're researching, scribble down any ideas that catch your eye as well as anything that doesn't appeal. Don't worry about crafting the perfect plan straight away. At the beginning it's more about collecting, sorting and collating the mountain of available information. You can edit and tidy things up later on.

Questions to consider

- **Where do I want to give birth?**
  You have a choice about where to have your baby. When considering this question, you should think about your health, your medical history, your pregnancy so far and the options available in your area.

  Midwife-led units, hospital, home or a private unit are possibilities. Talk to your doctor or midwife and visit the potential places, so you can weigh up the good and bad bits and come to the right decision for you and your baby.

- **Who do I want as my birth partner?**
  Most women like to have someone to support them during labour and childbirth. Many choose the father of the child, but that's not the only option. Anyone who gives you confidence can help. Friends, relatives or professionals like doulas (women whose job is to support another woman during the late stages of pregnancy, through childbirth and into the early days of motherhood) are all valid alternatives, or you may want to go it alone. It's about choosing what makes you most relaxed and comfortable.

- **Is there any special equipment I would like to try?**
  Birthing balls, beanbags, floor mats, birthing pools, TENS machines, soft music and aromatherapy oils can be used to help make the birthing process more personal and more bearable. Think about what you would like to try, and check whether it's available in the place you're planning to give birth. If not, make sure you buy or hire the equipment early so it's ready and waiting on the big day.

- **Do I have any particular preferences for the birth?**
  Some hospital or birthing units have special facilities available. These can include birthing pools, dedicated labour/delivery/recovery/postnatal rooms where you can stay in the same room throughout your stay and postnatal amenity side rooms that you can book for an overnight stay.

  Your doctor or midwife should tell you what's available and let you know the booking procedure. However, understand that birth is unpredictable and there's no guarantee the room will be free when your contractions start.

- **How would I prefer to be monitored?**
  Every baby is monitored throughout labour to make sure they are healthy and well. There are different ways of checking the baby's heartbeat to make sure there are no signs of distress. If everything is progressing well, the heart-beat may be checked every quarter of an hour or so with a Doppler device, or continually by a belt strapped around your waist. You can express a preference between these two options.

  However, problems, an epidural, a drip to strengthen contractions or any sign that your baby may be struggling can mean that continuous monitoring of your baby's heart using a clip attached to their scalp is necessary. In childbirth, safety should be the first consideration.

- **Would I like to move during labour?**
  Actively moving and participating in the process of labour can help labour progress, increase your feeling of control and boost confidence. However, it may make you a little tired, and sometimes moving around is not possible with standard epidurals.

- **Positions for labour and birth**
  The positions you adopt in labour can make a big difference to how it progresses. So experiment with positions like kneeling on all fours or leaning over a beanbag and think about what might work for you. Standing, sitting, squatting, lying, kneeling, doggy position or standing up, you can choose as many positions as you want and change whenever you feel the need.

- **What pain relief would I prefer?**
  In my experience, many women seem to adopt the 'suck it and see model' for pain relief and come into the delivery room with an open mind. You may prefer to try some of the less invasive methods of pain relief, like TENS, relaxation exercises and gas and air in the early stages, and then progress onto something stronger, such as an epidural, as and when you need it.

  Some women feel strongly about avoiding injectable medications, like pethidine, because they want to avoid that out of control and woozy feeling, while others love it. The choice is yours. List any you would consider and make a note of any strong preferences.

- **If my labour doesn't progress, what intervention would I prefer?**
  Sometimes labour doesn't progress as planned and needs a helping hand. This is called *augmentation of labour*. Your body has its own contraction hormone called oxytocin. If your contractions start to fade, or if they need a boost, you can be given an artificial version of oxytocin called Syntocinon, or your waters could be broken to speed things along. Consider

whether you would be happy to have this, or whether you would ideally prefer to wait and see what happens.

- **What are my feelings about instrumental delivery?**
  Very few women plan to have an assisted delivery, but sometimes things go wrong and babies need a little extra help into the world. You can say whether you have particular feelings about ventouse over forceps delivery and whether you would like a planned episiotomy to prevent tearing. You can also express whether you would like your partner to remain in the room if you need an assisted delivery.

  If you express a preference, your healthcare team will try to follow your wishes if possible. However, it is important to try to be adaptable to ensure the safe delivery of your baby. If you are worried, chat through your concerns with your healthcare team.

- **How do I feel about Caesarean sections?**
  A Caesarean section is an operation where an obstetric surgeon makes a cut in your abdomen and womb and removes your baby through it. It can be performed as a planned operation or in an emergency. If is carried out under epidural or spinal anaesthetic, you will be awake for the operation and your partner can stay with you.

- **How do I feel about an episiotomy?**
  An episiotomy is a small cut made in the perineum during birth. It done to avoid more extensive tearing, especially involving the structures surrounding the back passage. It may also be performed to help make the delivery of your baby a little easier, especially if you have an assisted delivery or a breech birth.

- **Do I have any preferences about clamping and cutting the cord?**
  If you'd like your partner to cut the cord or you'd prefer to delay the clamping of the cord, detail it in your plan. If everything goes well, the doctor or midwife delivering your little one should aim to help this happen.

- **Do I want an injection to be given to speed up the delivery of the placenta in the third stage?**
  Most hospitals and birth centres recommend an actively managed third stage of labour using an injection of a synthetic version of oxytocin. Research shows that this decreases the risk of losing lots of blood after the birth. However, you can choose to have a natural third stage, if you would prefer less intervention.

- **Do I want my baby delivered straight onto my body, or cleaned and wrapped first?**
  In the past, babies were often washed, wiped and returned to the mum as a neat little bundle wrapped in a blanket. You may prefer this, as newborn babies can be a little mucky. However, you may prefer immediate skin-to-skin contact to help with bonding and establishing breastfeeding.

- **Do I want my baby to be given an injection of vitamin K after the birth to prevent bleeding problems?**
  Babies have low levels of vitamin K at birth. For a small number of babies this can put them in danger of life-threatening haemorrhage. Because of this risk, it is recommended that all babies receive vitamin K after birth to protect them. The most effective way of giving this is by a single injection into the muscle of your baby's leg immediately after birth. An alternative is oral vitamin K, three doses are needed if your baby is breastfed. Two are given in the first week followed by a top-up when they are one-month old. Bottle-fed

babies only need two doses of vitamin K during their first week of life. The problem with this is that often doses can be missed in the chaos of the early weeks, which could put your baby at risk. You don't have to consent to the vitamin K injection. Talk to your doctor or midwife about your choice.

- **How am I planning to feed my baby?**
  Whether you're going to breast or formula feed, it's important to let your midwife know your plans so they can help you get things started after the birth.

- **Do I have any special requirements for the birth?**
  Everyone has different needs and demands during birth. Whether English is not your first language, you have special educational needs, you follow a specific diet or you have religious customs you'd like observed, this is the place to detail your individual needs. It will help your healthcare team help you to achieve a happy and healthy birth experience.

I had a great birth plan! Lots of careful thought and preparation in the months leading up to the birth. I had candles, oils, yoga balls and numerous different music playlists at the ready. I had my first contraction as I walked through the door of the hospital and was howling within seconds. The midwife asked, 'Have you thought about pain relief?' I growled, 'Give me an epidural!' And do you know what? It was the best thing. As soon as it was administered I completely relaxed and actually began to enjoy the whole experience. No doubt it was still intense but I was completely coherent and with it when my little man was born. I could still feel the contractions, move my legs and had the urge to push, nor did it slow the labour down! Listen to your body!

~ Sarah, Larne

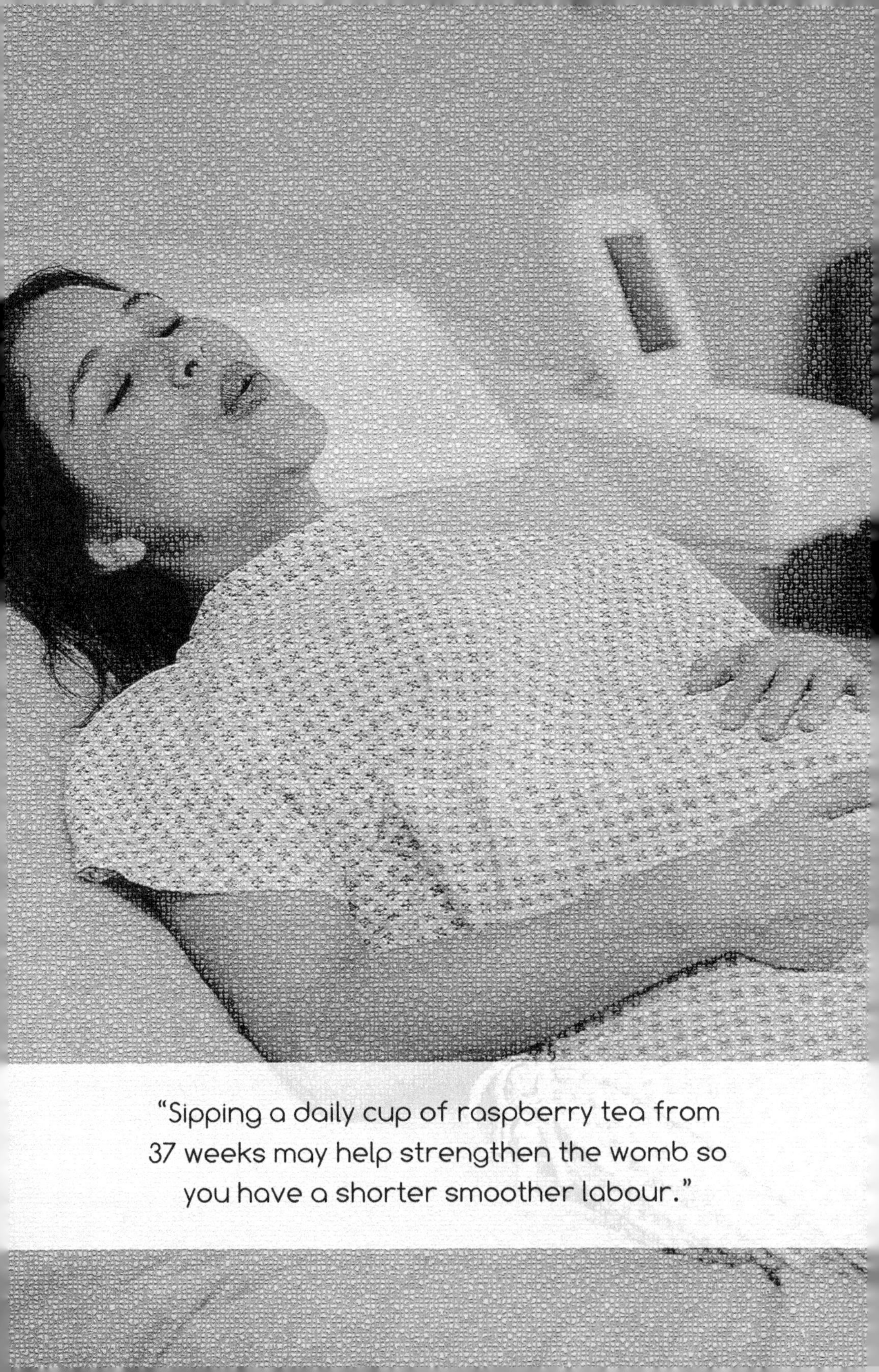

"Sipping a daily cup of raspberry tea from 37 weeks may help strengthen the womb so you have a shorter smoother labour."

44

HOW CAN I BRING LABOUR ON?

If only I had a pound for every time I'd been asked this question! Believe me, I'd be a very wealthy obstetrician. Lots of women are thoroughly frustrated and fed-up of pregnancy when they reach the end of the third trimester. They feel heavy, uncomfortable and impatient to meet their new baby.

Frequently I've been begged for techniques to bring on labour. In general, I'm a believer in waiting for nature to take its course. However, there are a few tricks you can try. I'm not making any promises, though. In my experience, babies tend to make their appearance when they're good and ready!

> *I had totally had enough of pregnancy when I got near term. I hated feeling so heavy and slow and I suppose the truth is, I'm very impatient and I was desperate to have my baby.*
>
> *I tried it all sex, raspberry leaf tea, curry. All the curry left me with was horrible indigestion that kept me up all night. I went into labour the morning after a Mexican meal, was it the chili or a coincidence? I don't know, I was glad to get it over and done with though!*
>
> **~ Jane, Leeds**

Get moving

Stay upright and active. It'll encourage your baby to move down into the pelvis and keep your blood pumping around the body. Don't overdo it, though. You need to rest too, so you're ready and raring to go when labour starts. If you're looking for exercise inspiration, check out my exercises to help manoeuvre your baby into the perfect position for birth.

Get fruity

Struggling to get your five a day? Add a little fruit to your diet and you may do a little more than improve your nutrition. A small study showed that eating six dates a day towards the end of pregnancy could encourage your cervix to ripen. I think it needs more research before I'm convinced by the evidence—but even if you don't go into labour, the dates should keep your bowels regular!

If dates aren't to your taste, pick a pineapple. They contain an enzyme called bromelain, which is also thought to soften the cervix. You'd need to eat an awful lot—but if you're desperate...

Tea time

Raspberry leaf tea is a type of herbal infusion that is packed with vitamins, minerals and tannins. It's popular with expectant mums because supping it late in pregnancy is thought to act as a uterine tonic. It has been used since the sixth century to strengthen the muscles of the womb, bring on labour and speed up delivery. Those are big expectations for a herbal brew, so does it really work?

Does raspberry leaf tea help?

Raspberry leaf is rich in micronutrients, including vitamins, minerals and a chemical called *fragine*. This is the ingredient thought to help strengthen and tone the uterine muscles, so they can work better in the second stage of labour.

Raspberry leaf tea may also help your womb shrink back to size after delivery and prevent bleeding after the birth.

Researchers have shown that red raspberry leaf tea daily may help strengthen the myometrium, shorten labour and reduce complications. There was also an indication that artificial rupture of the membranes, assisted deliveries and Caesarean sections may be slightly reduced. The differences weren't dramatic. but it could be something to consider, when you're reaching the end of pregnancy and desperate for delivery.

Care and cautions

For some people drinking raspberry leaf tea may not be a good thing. Chat to your doctor or midwife and stay off the pink stuff if:

- You're overdue (the stronger contractions could lead to distress in your baby)
- You've previously had a Caesarean section
- You have a Caesarean planned in this pregnancy
- You had premature labour in a previous pregnancy
- You've had bleeding or spotting in the last half of pregnancy
- You've had quick labours previously, especially if one lasted less than three hours

Raspberry leaf tea is an active substance, so don't take it before 37 weeks and don't down it by the bucket-load. Stick to no more than three cups a day. Try starting with one cup a day and gradually build up to two or three daily cuppas.

The spice of life

Lots of women swear that a curry kicked off contractions for them. The spices are meant to stimulate the bowel, which can trigger contractions. In my experience, it's as likely to keep you up all night groaning with indigestion or the trots, but if you really fancy a bhuna or a balti , tuck in.

Sexual healing

Sex started this whole adventure and maybe sex can bring it to a finale. Lots of women tell me that sex seemed to trigger labour for them. That could make some scientific sense, if your body is already ready and gearing up for labour. Semen contains chemicals called prostaglandins that can soften the cervix and make it ready to open up, so if you're both in the mood, it's worth a try.

Nipple stimulation

And while we're on the subject of sex, a little nipple action can also help release hormones that could trigger labour. And even if it doesn't work, it could get you in the mood for some action in between the sheets, double the benefits!

Party games

Having a baby shower? Well, make sure you have plenty of balloons. The action of blowing them up is meant to increase the pressure in the abdomen to get labour going—hopefully not before you've opened your pressies, though.

A helping hand

For the best way of bringing on birth, you'll need the help of a medical professional. A membrane sweep can bring on labour within twenty-four hours in fifty per cent of women.

What is a membrane sweep?

A membrane sweep isn't an extreme form of tidying up, as part of the urge to nest. Instead it's a drug free way of helping labour start. If you're reaching the end of your pregnancy and the end of your tether, a sweep can make you more likely to go into labour naturally, without the need for induction.

A sweep is a type of vaginal examination. Your doctor or midwife can assess the ripeness of your cervix and will use their fingers to make a circular movement around the opening of the neck of the womb. This sweeps the membranes surrounding the baby, separating them from the cervix. This separation releases natural hormones called prostaglandins, which may stimulate contractions and kick-start your labour.

Some women find a sweep a little uncomfortable and you may notice some painful tightening afterwards, or a little vaginal bleeding and mucous. They can all signal that labour may be imminent.

Where and when?

A sweep really is pretty quick and easy, like a normal vaginal examination. It will be done at your usual antenatal clinic, usually when you are overdue and ready for your baby to arrive.

Does it work?

After a sweep, there is a fifty/fifty chance that labour will start within the next twenty-four hours. If there's still no sign of things getting going, you can have a repeat sweep, or you may be offered a date for induction. Time to check your phone's charged and your bag's packed. Hopefully, it won't be long now!

Exercises to get your baby into a good position for birth

The perfect position for your baby's delivery is head down and with the back of the head towards the front of your tummy, which is known as the anterior position. Evidence shows that this can help make your labour a little shorter and easier. That has to be a good thing, doesn't it?

The good news is that most babies manage to get into this position towards the end of pregnancy. But if your little one is determined to stay breech or back-to-back, there are ways of coaxing them into place.

Your baby's back is heavier than the front, so gravity will ensure it naturally moves towards the lowest bit of your abdomen. Make the most of that fact, by trying out positions in which you lean forward. You can start these exercises from 34 weeks in your first pregnancy or 37 weeks if you've given birth before.

The scrubber

OK, this one is better than it sounds. It uses the time-tested floor-scrubbing position. Getting down on all fours can help you take deeper breaths and may also help to encourage your baby into the heads down position as well as moving it anterior. If you're getting an urge to nest, it can also ensure your floors are sparkling clean too. The perfect way to multi-task!

The Sally Bowles

Try sitting backwards on an upright chair, like Liza Minnelli in Cabaret to try to beat the breech. You can lean forward onto the back of the chair and watch the telly. Or why not rest a book or magazine on the chair back, so you can catch up on some reading?

The bum bounce

Say goodbye to the sofa and instead get yourself comfy kneeling on the floor. Lean forward and rest your body on cushions, a bean bag or a padded footstool. Try wiggling or swaying your hips to encourage your little one to get moving.

The angry pussy

It sounds weird, but it works, so get on your hands and knees and channel your inner moggy. Kneel on all fours, and slowly arch your back like a cat. Hold this for ten seconds and slowly release down.

This is a classic yoga position called the cat stretch. Try repeating it ten times.

Positions to avoid

Don't forget that if exercises can manipulate your baby's presentation to your benefit, they can also help encourage a less favourable position, so take care. In particular, try to avoid:

- Long journeys leaning back in seats, take a cushion so you're pitched a little forward.
- Lying on your back. Chilling out is good but relaxing back can encourage the wrong position and squash the big vein in your abdomen. Instead try lying on your side.
- Deep squats. To be honest, this kind of activity may be a physical impossibility late in pregnancy, unless you're pretty agile. Don't be tempted to experiment, though. It may cause your baby's head or bottom to engage before they've turned into a better position.

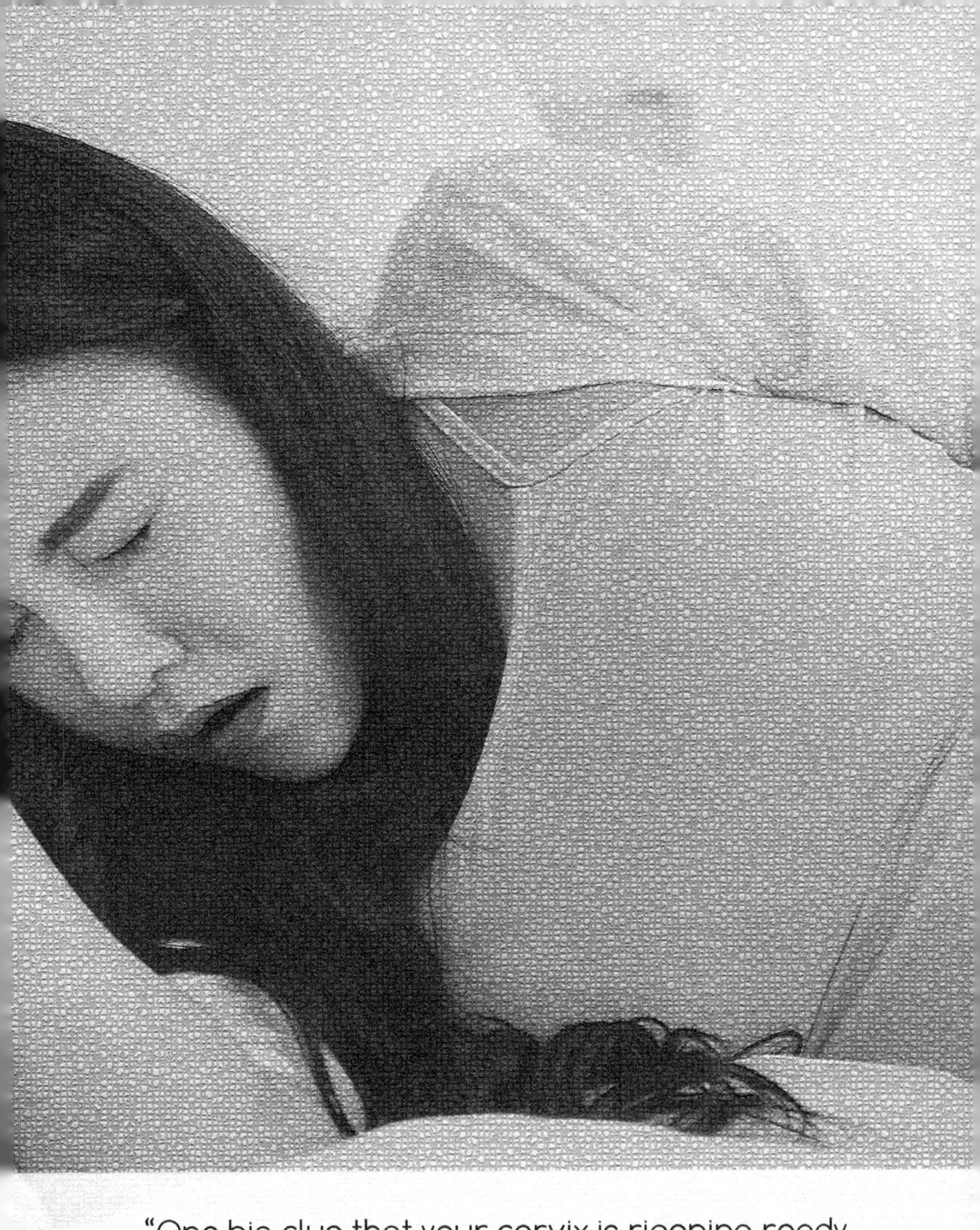

"One big clue that your cervix is ripening ready for the birth is seeing a 'show' of mucous discharge, streaked with blood."

45

HOW CAN I TELL THE DIFFERENCE BETWEEN FALSE AND TRUE LABOUR?

For forty long weeks, your body and your baby have both been building up to this moment. But the question is, will you know when you're really in labour? It can be tricky to tell, particularly if this is your first baby. There's probably been a number of times in the past few days and weeks when pain and pressure have made you wonder if labour has started. But don't panic, I've got the key clues so you don't get caught by surprise.

Real or false labour?

It's a big job propelling your baby into the world. To get good and ready, your womb prepares by practising a little. These practice tightenings of the muscles of the uterus are called Braxton Hicks contractions, after the doctor who first described them back in 1872.

They're usually irregular and pretty infrequent and can be uncomfortable but shouldn't cause severe pain. They start early on in pregnancy but only become strong enough to feel from around the twenty-eighth week. More women feel them towards the end of pregnancy, as the body is counting down to the big day.

Is it Braxton Hicks or labour?

Braxton Hicks contractions don't follow a regular pattern; they tend to come and go. You may trigger them if you're really active and running around, if your bladder is full, when you're dehydrated or if you have sex. They won't increase in frequency and intensity the way labour contractions do. If you rest quietly, or change position, they often die away.

What should you do?

If you've already reached 37 weeks and feel well, you don't need to do anything. If you're in discomfort, try sipping water to increase hydration, lie on your left-hand side or have a relaxing bath.

If it's before term and you're worried that you're in labour, get in touch with your doctor, midwife or maternity unit. They may arrange some tests to monitor the baby and record the frequency and duration of your contractions. Sometimes they may also do an internal examination to check for other signs of labour, like dilation of your cervix.

Early indications of labour

In the early stages of labour, you may not notice many symptoms but inside your body changes may be afoot.

- **Cervical change**

  During pregnancy, your cervix is long, firm, closed and sealed with a plug of mucous.

  It's positioned pointing to the back of your vagina. In late pregnancy, it gets ready to open up in labour. It moves nearer to the front of your vagina and gets softer and flatter. This process is called effacement. It can happen days or just hours before delivery. Many women are unaware that this is occurring, although you may feel backache, tummy ache or some mild regular contractions.

- **Show**

  One big clue that your cervix is ripening is seeing a 'show' of mucous discharge, streaked with blood. This is the plug of mucous that has been protecting the entrance to the womb for the past nine months. It was created from around seven weeks to seal the neck of the womb and prevent any infections penetrating and harming your baby.

  It stays in place as your womb's built-in bug barrier until your cervix starts to soften and shorten during the first stage of labour.

What is mucous?

You've probably used the word mucous to describe snot from your nose, or slime if you're suffering from diarrhoea. It's a slippery substance made by the cells that line your nose, lungs, gut and vagina. It can be thin and slimy or thick and gloopy, and our bodies produce it in bucket loads. Our noses alone pour out a litre a day.

Show time

The plug may be shed in one big, jelly-like blob, or you may simply notice a thicker, increased discharge. It can be clear or cloudy and pink or brown stained from the blood. This is your signal that your body is primed for the birth.

When will the baby come?

Seeing a show doesn't mean that labour is imminent. Active labour starts when your waters break or you get painful, regular contractions. The mucous is simply a sign that the cervix is starting to open. If you've had a baby before, labour can sometimes follow rapidly. However, if it's your first time you may have another week or so to wait.

What should you do?

There's no need to call your midwife when you have a show, although if you're bleeding heavily or you're worried you're going into labour too early, contact your maternity unit straight away. Otherwise, it's time to check your bag, get some rest and get ready, your baby may soon be on their way.

- **Diarrhoea**

  Late on in pregnancy, loose bowel movements together with a little nausea or vomiting, can be an early signal that you're going into labour. It's your body's way of clearing the route through the pelvis for your baby.

- **Mood change**

  During the latent phase of labour, you (or your partner) may notice that you're a bit more emotional, excitable and easily upset or moody. If this is your only symptom it's probably safe to put off calling the midwife for a little while.

- **Aches and pains**

  You will probably notice a dull pain in your back that comes on at regular intervals. This can spread around to your lower abdomen, a bit like crampy period pains.

It's looking like labour:

- **Regular painful contractions**

  Doctor, midwives and baby books talk about regular contractions, but what does that mean? I say that we should refer to frequent and strong contractions as the important symptom of labour. In fact, I can usually tell when someone is in labour over the phone because they can't talk properly when a contraction comes due to the pain.

  If your contractions are painful, lasting twenty seconds to a minute, and are coming every five to seven minutes (or even more frequently) you might well be into the active stage of labour. If that's the case, you don't need to sit there with a stop clock. You can call your doctor, midwife or the labour ward now.

- **A gush or a trickle of fluid from the vagina**

  You may have seen images in films, or heard stories of women's water breaking in a massive gush in the centre of the supermarket or train station. The truth is that most women's waters actually break during labour at the height of a contraction. However, it can sometimes happen before active contractions start. That can be at home, in the car or, of course, in the supermarket.

  Inside your womb your baby grows and develops inside a bag of fluid called the amniotic sac. It cushions and protects them from any bumps and bangs. When your baby is ready to make their entry into the world, the bag bursts and the fluid escapes through your vagina. Your waters have broken. The liquid can come as a little trickle or as a full-on flood. Many women think that they may be wetting themselves, but unlike the stream of urine you're totally unable to control the flow of amniotic fluid.

Which water?

Amniotic fluid is clear and a pale straw-like colour. Sounds familiar? The truth is your waters can look a lot like wee, so it can be difficult to tell them apart. The clue is that the waters come out of your vagina, not the hole in front so it may feel rather damp and watery at the entrance. It's sensible to keep a pad and towel handy to spare any mess and blushes.

The waters should not be smelly, dark or discoloured. A pink tinge at the beginning is normal, but clear and obvious bleeding or green, black or brown staining is not. Sometimes, if your baby is having difficulties or is distressed they may open their bowels and pass meconium when they are still in the womb. Contact your healthcare team immediately if you notice any problem, as you and your baby may need urgent medical help.

What should I do?

If you're having regular contractions and your waters have broken naturally, it's time to contact your doctor or midwife, call your partner and check your bag is ready and packed. It shouldn't be long until you meet your baby. Exciting times lie ahead!

If your waters break before labour starts, known as pre-labour rupture of membranes **(PROM)**, pop a pad in to catch the flow and phone your doctor, midwife or the labour ward for advice. Without the protective fluid surrounding them, your baby could be at risk of infection. Labour is likely to start spontaneously within twenty-four hours. However, if it doesn't, inducing labour may be recommended.

Remember, if you're worried and unsure, get in touch with the delivery unit. They can give you advice, guidance and some friendly reassurance. Don't worry if you need to go in for a check-up, only to be examined by a doctor or midwife, and sent home again. They'll be used to uncertain mums. False labour contractions have an annoying way of disappearing the moment you step onto the labour ward. It's sod's law and women often feel embarrassed—but really it's not a problem. You can pop back home again, get some rest and wait until your little one is ready to make their grand entrance.

I am a midwife myself and felt pretty safe during my pregnancy. My waters broke at 37+2 and I didn't realise at first, it was just a trickle. I had a normal pregnancy check-up booked that day anyway, and my consultant examined me and looked a bit surprised when I had already a cervix opening of 4 cm. When I turned up at the hospital I was feeling 'funny.' No contractions yet, but 5cm now! But soon I started to feel the contractions. OMG! I could not have missed these!

~ Kristina, London

What to do when labour starts

It's been a nine month wait to meet your baby and you've probably been ticking off the days and analysing every tightening and twinge. Well, the big moment is here. Your contractions are regular and getting stronger, so what should you do now?

Don't panic!

The most important thing to do is to stay calm. Your body was designed for this and despite the scare stories about babies appearing at lightning speed down the loo or in the taxi, it's much more likely you'll have plenty of time before your little one arrives.

Partner on call

Get in touch with your birth partner, so they know they could be called into action at any moment.

Put the hospital bag by the door

Whether you packed it months ago, or left it to the last minute, now you need to make sure you've got everything you need for labour, birth and beyond. Check that your hand-held notes, your birth plan and your list of contact numbers are close at hand, and charge your phone so it's ready if you need it.

Measure and monitor

It's time to rock out the stopwatch function on your phone. Time the length and frequency of your contractions, so you can let your midwife know.

Call the carers

If you have other children, you should get in contact with the friend, family or babysitter who's going to look after them while you're otherwise engaged. Pretty soon they may be meeting a new little brother or sister.

Call the professionals

If you're not sure whether it's labour, you're worried, or you'd like a little advice, phone your midwife or the labour ward. This is particularly important if you're having a home birth, so your midwife is aware and can make plans.

Some centres recommend waiting until your contractions are five minutes apart, I'd say that you should see how you feel and never be afraid to ask for support and guidance. If you do want to go into the labour ward, or birth centre, it's important to phone first so they know to expect you. Now's the time to wish you good luck—there's not long to wait.

Mum's conundrum

I read somewhere that the latent phase of labour can last for days, which sounds horrible. What is the latent phase of labour and how can I survive it?

~ Hannah, Cardiff

Dr Keith says:

You may have seen the term latent labour in books or blogs and thought, surely you're in labour or you're not? Actually, it's not as cut and dried as that. Before you go into labour your cervix needs to transform from a long, firm tube into a soft, flat, squishy circle.

The National Institute for Health and Care Excellence (NICE) defines active labour as:

'The presence of regular painful contractions together with progressive dilatation of the cervix from 4cm.'

As you can see, there can be quite a bit of cervical change without being officially in active labour. That's the latent phase. In the weeks preceding labour, the neck of the womb gradually becomes shorter, flatter and softer in a process known as effacement. For that to happen, you'll need lots of contractions. Let's go back to those nice people at NICE. They define the latent phase as:

'A period of time that is not necessarily continuous, when there are painful contractions together with some cervical change, including cervical effacement and dilatation up to 4 cm.'

You can be in this early stage for a long time before things really get going. The experience of the latent phase can vary hugely between women. You may notice pains, tightenings and back ache, or you may have little significant discomfort.

Early pains

The pains may start in your back and then develop into crampy discomfort, a little like period pains. These cramps can build into contractions, but unlike full-blown labour there may not be a regular pattern and they can come and go. As well as the contractions, you may notice a show of blood and mucous in your knickers, that's the sign your cervix is changing and things are definitely getting going.

It can be dispiriting if you are in pain for a long time, without properly progressing into labour, but there's lots you can do to ease the discomfort and help yourself:

- You've got a busy and exhausting time ahead, so make sure you allow yourself plenty of time to rest and relax.
- Drink plenty of fluids to stay hydrated and eat regular snacks and meals so you're fuelled for labour.
- Empty your bladder every couple of hours, even if you don't feel the need. It can help things along.
- Water can soothe and support your body, so try a warm bath.
- If your back is aching, it's time for your partner to practise their back-massage technique.
- Paracetamol is a pretty effective painkiller and can really help with discomfort in the latent phase. Take 1g (usually two tablets) no more than every four hours, and make sure you don't take more than four doses in twenty-four hours.
- You've probably used a hot water bottle or wheat bag for period pains, well, now's the time to dig it out again and use it to soothe your aching back.
- If you hired or bought a ***TENS machine***, put it to use. It can help with the pain of early labour.

46

WHAT HAPPENS IF LABOUR NEEDS TO BE INDUCED?

Usually, labour will start spontaneously, but in as many as one in five pregnancies it needs a helping hand to kick-start the process. This is known as induction of labour; it will be offered if your doctor and midwife believe it is the safest thing for you and your baby.

Why would I be induced?

Your healthcare team will suggest an induction if it is in the best interests of your baby. It can be a lot to take in, but your doctor or midwife should talk you through their reasons as well as helping you weigh up the pros and cons. Feel free to ask any questions about your worries and concerns, and be reassured that no one will do anything to which you haven't consented.

If your baby is late: The most common reason for inducing labour is because a baby is overdue. A few days don't usually matter, but the longer you go over, the greater the danger that the placenta can deteriorate. This can really affect your baby's health, so your labour may need to be brought on when you go seven to ten days past your due date.

If your waters break before labour starts: This is known as pre-labour rupture of membranes (PROM). Without the protective fluid surrounding them, your baby could be at risk of infection. Labour usually starts spontaneously within twenty-four hours, however, if it doesn't, your midwife may recommend an induction.

If you decline induction, waiting for contractions to start after twenty-four hours can double your baby's risk of getting an infection. However, you can choose to closely monitor the movements, fluid and temperature while you wait to go into labour naturally. Even if you have no signs of infection and go into labour naturally more than twenty-four hours after your waters have broken, a hospital birth will be recommended in case your baby needs a little extra help after delivery. If your waters have been broken for over forty-eight hours, the risk of infection to you and your baby increases. It really is important to get your baby delivered quickly.

For health and wellbeing: Sometimes you or your baby may develop a problem, which means it is safer to get on with delivery. This could be because you have pre-eclampsia or other health problems, or your baby may be not growing and developing well, and so would be better off out of the womb.

What happens during induction?

There are a number of ways of kick-starting contractions. The method used will depend on how urgent it is to deliver your baby and how ripe and ready your cervix is. In general, the process isn't painful, although it may be uncomfortable. Once induction has started, you'll have to stay in hospital, so you can be checked and monitored. It can often take a while, so make sure you pack plenty of books and magazines to while away the time.

Initially, you may be offered a sweep of the membranes, which I described in the section on kicking off labour. It's a type of vaginal examination that can use the fingers to assess the ripeness of your cervix and gently sweep the membranes surrounding your baby, separating them from your cervix. This separation releases prostaglandins, which may stimulate the start of labour. If that doesn't do the trick, your midwife or doctor may try some other measures:

Pessary

Your body produces prostaglandins, but there are also medications available that contain similar chemicals. Your midwife can put a gel or pessary containing these into your vagina. It helps to ripen the cervix so it softens and shortens. It can also trigger tightenings, but don't expect instant drama. The effect isn't immediate and you may need a couple of doses before your body starts to respond.

Syntocinon drip

Your body has its own contraction hormone, called oxytocin. When you're induced, you may be offered an artificial version of oxytocin called Syntocinon. It's given by a drip and works immediately to make your contractions stronger and more frequent. However, they can also be intense, so you may find you need extra pain relief, like an epidural.

Artificial rupture of the membranes

If your cervix has already ripened and started to dilate, your midwife or doctor can do an internal examination and break your waters with a small hook.

What if it doesn't work?

Sometimes all the sweeps, pessaries and drips simply don't do the job. If induction doesn't get labour going, you might be offered a Caesarean section.

Every woman feels different. Some have had enough of pregnancy when they reach term and are delighted to accept an induction.

Others are upset by the over-medicalisation of their birth. If that's you, try not to dwell on the negatives. I've delivered many induced babies, so I've seen that the births can be a great experience too. The most important thing is that you'll have a wonderful, healthy baby at the end of it. Talk to your midwife and doctor about your concerns and good luck for the adventure ahead.

I was induced at ten days over my due date. I was given the pessary on Sunday afternoon and on Monday morning I was given a paracetamol and told to get dressed and walk around the hospital car park!

I started contracting every minute and a half, with each contraction lasting for a minute. I couldn't have got through this without my TENS machine which was cranked right up. I found this a great comfort as it gave me something to concentrate on and have a little control amidst the pain.

I was later given diamorphine and had a warm bath, which helped a little. After failure to progress, I was given the oxytocin drip in conjunction with an epidural. Before the epidural catheter was put in place, the anaesthetist asked me my pain level on a scale of one to ten. I wanted to say ten, but trying to be brave said eight and a half. After the epidural, he asked me the same thing. The relief was instant. I remember saying, 'Six. No, four. No, one...' I felt nothing! My legs were like someone else's stretched out in front of me, and the only way I could tell if I was having a contraction was when my tummy went hard.

After so much pain for a sustained period of time, it was great to suddenly feel nothing—but strange and a bit of an anti-climax to be numb when it came to the actual birth. In the end, I had an episiotomy (for which I was grateful I couldn't feel anything) and with the assistance of ventouse suction, my beautiful little girl was born on Tuesday morning weighing 7.6lbs.

~ Kate, Haslemere

47

WILL I BE ABLE TO COPE WITH THE PAIN OF LABOUR?

Lots of women are frightened about the prospect of pain in labour and scare stories from friends and family members who've given birth definitely don't help. In many ways, human childbirth is strange; the baby's head is bigger than the mother's pelvis, so delivery can be a challenge. Most other mammals don't experience the sort of pain that humans suffer, because they don't have this physical restriction. But remember that women have been giving birth since the beginning of time, so it can be done. Whether you go into a zen-like trance or whoop and holler, you'll find your own way of coping. Be reassured, that if the pain becomes too much for you to deal with, there are many pain-killing options to provide relief.

It's good to know about potential pain-relief before the birth, so you understand the pros and cons. You may feel that you have a clear idea about the pain relief you definitely want and don't want. Remember that in the heat of labour, your plans and preferences might change. Do what feels best for you at the time and don't feel guilty or upset if you opt for something that wasn't on your birth plan.

Medical management like epidurals, gas and air and injectable drugs like pethidine can be effective—but I'm also a big believer in the power of the mind and I've seen methods like hypnotherapy, breathing exercises and relaxation make a big difference to the way women experience and cope with pain. In this section, I will talk about the natural approaches to overcoming pain, which can be incredibly helpful especially towards the beginning of labour.

The natural approach

In the centuries before modern medications and epidurals, women relied on relaxation, breathing and distraction techniques to help them cope with pain. Tricks and tips were handed down from mother to daughter. These methods can still be useful and effective today. And the good news is, they're side-effect free.

Breathing and relaxation

When you are tense and anxious, you feel more pain. So whatever pain relief you are planning, it can help to learn to relax through contractions. It will help you manage labour better and can be fantastic during the early stages.

Most antenatal classes will go over basic breathing techniques and show you exercises to help you learn to relax. The trick is to breathe slowly and rhythmically, focusing on the air going in and out. This concentration and control can distract you from the tightenings in your tummy and can actually make them hurt less too.

Hypnobirthing

The human brain is incredibly powerful; mind really can gain control over matter. Our emotions, experiences and moods can have a huge impact on the way we experience pain. Hypnobirthing taps into this power and can help you achieve a birth that is calmer, more natural and less painful.

Self-hypnosis builds on natural relaxation techniques. When you prepare for the birth with hypnosis, you work to replace your feelings of anxiety and fear with the expectation of a safe, comfortable birth.

Because of this, you'll be more relaxed in labour, which can actually help prevent pain. Tense muscles hurt more and when you're stressed you'll release lots of adrenaline which stops your body producing the feel-good hormones endorphins. So if you're laid back, your pain will be too.

What is hypnosis?

Hypnosis is a state of deep relaxation. When in this state, you can focus intensely on a single thought or feeling and you may be more open to suggestions that can change your behaviour or relieve your symptoms. Hypnosis has been shown in research to help prevent anxiety in pregnancy and to relieve pain during labour and birth.

DIY

Self-hypnosis can be particularly useful in the delivery suite. It can be achieved by a combination of breathing techniques, deep relaxation exercises and visualising a positive labour and delivery. You'll also learn about the physical facts of childbirth and precisely what is happening to your body at each stage. If you understand the process, it's easier to let go of your fears. This is reinforced with plenty of positive thoughts and language.

If you expect a good birth experience, you're more likely to get a good birth experience. With less stress, anxiety and fear you should feel more calm and in control. Research suggests that women who use hypnosis in labour may need less pain relief and fewer epidurals.

Gail Johnson, from the Royal College of Midwives, said that women should not worry about their preconceived ideas of hypnosis, such as losing control of their body or being unable to remember the birth.

It's not one, two, three, go into a trance and wake up with a baby.

The self-hypnosis process is often less about being in a trance and more about focusing on something other than pain. Classes are available in many hospitals and clinics across the country, with lots of independent midwives offering hypnosis along with more traditional pain control techniques. Johnson emphasised:

It's important that women are confident the people running the courses are competent and they seek out reputable trainers, but we think anything which offers women a wider choice in their pain relief is good. We're not saying it's right for all women, it's part of a wider spectrum of support and care for women.

I can't tell you that hypnobirthing will give you the perfect natural birth. I've seen women who have found it wonderfully effective and empowering and others who have quickly screamed for more drugs. However, it can be an interesting and useful way to gain control over your body, learn relaxation and harness the power of the mind, which has to be useful not just for birth but for life beyond.

I was amazed at the difference between my first birth and my second. In my first pregnancy, I was much more prepared. I had practised the relaxation techniques, the yoga breathing and a bit of meditation. During the birth, I found it was incredible. When I kept calm and breathed with each contraction, the feelings and contractions were intense but manageable. But as soon as I forgot to concentrate, it was overwhelmingly painful and—dare I say—a bit frightening. Luckily, I mostly managed to stay focused.

I was much less prepared for my second birth: I hadn't had a chance to get all zen, hadn't been to yoga and didn't feel so confident or ready. Would I remember how to breathe? Not really, was the answer and I found it much harder to keep the pain under control.

~ Lara, Chichester

Complementary therapies

We know that anxiety can increase the perception of pain, so any treatment that relaxes and empowers you may provide some relief. For this reason, complementary therapies are becoming increasingly popular in childbirth. Whether it's acupuncture or aromatherapy, the treatments may soothe discomfort and help you have a positive experience of labour and birth.

The essential oils of aromatherapy, stimulation of the energy channels in acupuncture and acupressure, or the power of touch in reflexology and massage can aid relaxation decrease stress and ease pain.

For some techniques, you can do-it-yourself, or rely on your birth partner for a helping hand. For other therapies, it's better to consult with a qualified practitioner with experience in the care of pregnant women. Chat to your doctor or midwife. They may have experience with some therapies, or they may be happy for your therapist to accompany you in labour so you can work together to achieve a great birth experience.

Birth ball

A birth ball is a bit like those big bouncy globes that you may have seen at the gym. It's a good way of exploring different labour positions, opening the pelvis and easing lower back pain. You can kneel and lean over the ball, or sit on it and gently bounce or rotate your hips. The movement can be soothing and the activity can be a good distraction from contractions.

They may be available in your labour unit, so check with your midwife. However, they are also widely available to buy at a pretty reasonable price. They're useful for exercises to strengthen the core muscles after the birth, too.

Water birth

For thousands of years, women have instinctively used water for soothing support in labour. Lots of pregnant mums find that being submerged in warm liquid, helps them relax, move more easily and deal with pain better.

Many hospitals have birth pools, or you can hire one to use at home. However, it's a good idea to talk to your midwife or doctor about your wishes early, so the necessary arrangements can be put in place. If you don't have a pool, you can still harness the wonder of water. Lots of mums find a warm bath can be relaxing and soothing, especially in the early stages of labour.

TENS machines (transcutaneous electrical nerve stimulation)

While this is definitely not natural, I've added it in this section because TENS can be a useful support in the early stages of labour.

A TENS machine may help with some of the discomfort when labour starts. It's a battery-powered device, which stimulates your nerves with low levels of electrical current. This is believed to trigger the body to produce endorphins, our built-in painkillers. It may also decrease the number of pain signals being sent to the brain.

It works on something called the gate theory for pain, by stimulating different sensory pathways you feel the pain less, like rubbing your leg when you bump it.

There may be machines available in your labour unit, or you can hire or buy one, so it's ready and waiting by the time labour begins. Practise with the device when you reach 37 weeks, so you know how to use it properly.

TENS works better if you start using it in early labour, especially in conjunction with breathing and relaxation techniques. It definitely can't be used in a birth pool—water and electricity are not a good combination!

> *I used a TENS machine for early contractions. I can't really say it helped with the pain but perhaps as a distraction it was useful. My hypnobirthing CD was helpful to relax during the last few weeks of pregnancy but I did not actually use any of the techniques during the birth. The midwives were great in helping with breathing and pushing.*
>
> ~ **Jennifer, London**

Screaming or silence, what's your labour preference?

I've delivered over three thousand babies and it can be a noisy process. Some women are utterly silent, while others can scream the house down. It's a matter of individual preference and pure animal instinct. And if you think that chatty women have noisy births, while shy retiring types remain quiet and reserved, you're wrong. It can be impossible to predict the wailers from the whisperers before you get down to the business end of the birth.

Grunts and groans

Making a noise isn't only an expression of pain or exertion, it can actually make pushing more effective. There's a reason those professional tennis players make grunting noises when they serve or make a heavy hit. If you exhale and make a noise with each exertion or push, it can make sure you keep breathing and add impetus to your effort.

Silence can be golden

However, you don't have to shout the ward down to deliver effectively. For some women, silent concentration can work brilliantly. I remember one lady who was terrified of what childbirth might entail. Having become pregnant unexpectedly, she was referred to me by a friend who had had a positive experience under my care. She said I was the answer to her fears.

When the day came, I think I was more afraid than she was: she had heaped her concerns and expectations on me, completely handing over responsibility for them. When I walked into her room, she barely acknowledged me and said, 'Get on with it!' During the procedure, she never said a word. She didn't respond when I asked her questions, and much of the time she appeared to be asleep, internalising absolutely everything. Her partner was concerned, understandably, about her being so unresponsive, but as soon as she was in the recovery area, with baby in her arms, she declared to me that childbirth was one of the best experiences of her life. The peaceful environment helped her stay calm and focused on the job in hand.

Here, mums have shared their experiences. They perfectly illustrate that there is no 'right' way to behave in labour, only the right way for you.

With my first labour, I was totally silent and it felt rather serene, that's the bliss of a good epidural. The second time it was a bit more painful and I screamed and hollered like a mad woman. I kept swearing during the contractions and then apologising to the midwife in between!

~ Jane, Leeds

I didn't make a noise at all in labour, I don't know why but pain makes me go quiet. It was the same when I broke my leg I kind of disappear into myself. I think it helps me cope.

~ Philippa, Gloucester

I've always been a bit of a shouter in labour, so much so that I noticed that the first thing my other half put in the hospital bag was noise-cancelling headphones!

~ Fi, Leeds

I didn't say much when I was pushing, to be honest, it was difficult to get a word in because my husband kept on encouraging me. I think I pushed harder to get a bit of peace!

~ Emma, London

I kept screaming and swearing in labour, then when the contraction faded, I was embarrassed and kept apologising.

~ Elizabeth, Swansea

48

WHAT PAIN RELIEF CAN I USE?

If the natural methods of pain relief in the last section are no longer enough, then modern medicine offers plenty of options to help ease the discomfort of labour and birth. However, don't get the idea that it's a case of choosing one or the other. All the techniques can be used as and when you need them, so you can have the best and most comfortable birth experience possible.

In early labour, it is really helpful to have a calm tranquil environment full of positive determined energy. Relaxation, self-hypnosis and movement can help you control your experience of the pain. For some women and some births this can be enough, but most women need something a little stronger as things progress.

I've said this before—but I think it's worth repeating yet again: try to stay open and flexible because labour is a dynamic process and things don't always go according to a fixed plan. The truth is, unless you have experienced labour before, you cannot really know how it will affect you. Even if this isn't your first delivery, each birth is different depending on the size and position of the baby.

Too many women feel guilty because they couldn't cope with pain and had analgesia that wasn't in their birth plan. The truth is, no one knows how they'll feel, so I'd recommend an adaptable approach to pain relief. The good news is, there are some effective options:

Gas and air

Gas and air, or to use its other name, Entonox, is the most popular method of pain relief in labour. Eight out of every ten women use it to help them cope with their contractions.

It is a colourless, odourless gas, made up of half laughing gas (nitrous oxide) and half oxygen to keep you alive. It used to be gas and air, hence the name, but we have now enriched the air with extra oxygen. You inhale it through a plastic mask or by biting on a mouthpiece so there is an airtight seal. The trick is to breathe it in as a contraction is starting so the relief is in place by the time the pain reaches a peak. In between contractions, you can stop taking the gas and air and the effects quickly fade.

The great thing about Entonox is that it works immediately. It doesn't kill the pain but it can take the edge off it and make it more bearable. It is good for early labour. Unfortunately, it can make some mothers feel sick and many women feel a little woozy and giggly, a bit like being drunk. Most mums tell me that this spaced-out feeling is better than screaming with pain.

Entonox is widely available for use at home, in a birth centre or in hospital and it can also be used when you're labouring in water.

Injectable pain relief in labour

Drugs like diamorphine, pethidine or meptazinol can be given by an injection into the muscles of your legs or bottom. Different hospitals tend to use differing medications, so chat to your midwife about the options available to you.

Although the specific medications vary in their actions and side-effects, they are all strong painkillers related to the drug opium, so they can decrease pain, help you relax and even allow you to get some sleep. The injections can make you feel a little spaced-out and drowsy. They can also cause nausea and vomiting, so you may need an anti-sickness injection at the same time. It is not safe to use the birthing pool for at least two hours after the injection.

The medications can cross the placenta into your baby's system, so they should not be given too close to the birth because your baby may be sluggish and slow to breathe after delivery. If this happens, the paediatrician will stimulate your baby and give them oxygen.

Epidural

An epidural is a blanket term for a regional anaesthetic placed in the lower back to block pain and sensation in the pelvis and legs. It's the gold standard for pain relief in labour, and really useful for giving mothers a break from labour pains so they can gather their strength for the delivery stage. It is always performed by an experienced anaesthetist and there are a few variations in the medication given and the way it is topped up. Your anaesthetist will help you decide on the best one for your particular individual circumstances in labour.

The amount of anaesthetic used and the level to which the area will be numbed will depend on your stage of labour. Less intense and extensive mobile epidurals are becoming increasingly popular, and later on in labour, it can help to have some sensation so you are able to push effectively.

Epidurals are an incredibly effective method of pain relief, without causing sedation or any change in awareness. It can also bring down blood pressure, which can be useful in women with pre-eclampsia. It will not affect your baby at all.

My first pregnancy I had gas and air at first and then an epidural, I felt so much more relaxed after having it and was waiting for the birth. Second pregnancy one puff of gas and air and she was out. I felt both experiences were good and were right at the time. I put on my birth plan to go with the flow as I know they don't always work out as planned.

~ Sam, Northfields

Are there any disadvantages with epidurals?

There are pros and cons to every method of pain relief. An epidural decreases the sensation from the pelvis down. That's great for pain relief, but it also means it can be impossible to move around and sometimes women need a catheter to drain their bladder. However, a number of hospitals (including mine) now offer new, mobile epidurals, which maintain some leg sensation and movement.

Because of the decreased sensation, some women struggle to push constructively. This can put them at increased risk of needing forceps or ventouse to help deliver the baby, but usually we can decrease the numbness towards the end to try to overcome this.

It's important to remember that any epidural can take time to put in. You need to wait for the anaesthetist, and it can be a bit of a fiddly procedure, so it could be three-quarters of an hour or so before the pain is eased. Sometimes the baby is too impatient to wait for the pain relief.

Many women are anxious about epidurals, but if we look at the evidence, the rate of complications is actually low, especially if you're being cared for by an experienced anaesthetist.

One of the most common problems is when there is a leak of the fluid that bathes the nerves. We call this a dural tap, and it happens about once in 200 times. The anaesthetist can usually tell when this happens because they see a leak of the spinal fluid at the time of the epidural. It can lead to a special kind of headache that is much worse when you get up and eases off when you lay down. It can settle on its own, but if it doesn't, it's easily curable. We take a little blood from the arm and use it to plug the gap in the epidural space. This is called a blood patch.

Sometimes epidurals only work on one side. If that happens, it can feel a little weird, but we can easily take the epidural catheter out and put another one in. However, the thing that women really worry about is neurological damage. Happily, this is very rare indeed. Minor neurological damage occurs about one in ten thousand times; that can be a little numb patch on the toe or thigh that goes away with time. Major neurological damage only happens 1.8 in 100,000 times, which is good odds and, I hope, a reassuring figure.

What happens when you have an epidural?

When an epidural is going to be inserted, firstly the anaesthetist will put a little drip into your arm to provide fluids. Then you'll be asked to sit up and curve your back outwards into the position that my anaesthetic colleague Dr Daryl Dob describes as being like a sulky teenager, this gives you a good idea of the exact pose to adopt! Sometimes, if it's more comfortable you can lie down on your side and curl up into a ball.

A little local anaesthetic is injected to numb your skin. This stings a little before the area goes numb, then the anaesthetist finds the fluid which bathes the nerves with a tiny needle and puts a low dose of local anaesthetic into the fluid, which gets rid of the contraction pains.

A small needle is used to access the epidural space (the outermost part of the spinal canal), then a narrow tube called a catheter is inserted to inject medication to decrease pain and feeling in the pelvis and legs. Often it can be set up so you can top up the pain relief according to your own needs.

There's an art to epidurals. It's about giving enough so the contractions can be felt but they're not painful.

49

WHAT ARE THE CHANCES I'LL NEED A CAESAREAN SECTION?

You probably already know what a Caesarean section is. It's so commonly done now, with around one in four pregnancies being delivered by a planned or emergency C-Section, that it is a familiar part of our language. Put simply, a Caesarean is an operation where an obstetric surgeon makes a cut in your abdomen and womb and removes your baby through it.

History of Caesareans

The first recorded surgical removal of a baby comes from ancient Chinese records. Luzhong, a sixth-generation descendant of the Yellow Emperor, who ruled way back in 2500 BCE, had six sons, all born by *cutting open the body*. A little later, in India in the third century BCE, it is recorded that the mother of Bindusara, the second emperor of India, accidentally consumed poison and died when she was close to delivering him. The story goes that Chanakya, the Chandragupta's teacher and adviser, cut open the belly of the queen and took out the baby, thus saving the baby's life.

What about Caesar?

But what about Julius Caesar? I hear you cry. Well, the truth is that the widely accepted assumption the Roman dictator was born by Caesarean section is probably untrue. His mother, Aurelia, successfully gave birth to her son and lived to see him become Emperor. At that time, they weren't as efficient as preventing bleeding and stitching the womb back together, so the operation was fatal. So it seems likely she had a safe, vaginal delivery.

However, in Latin the verb **caesus** means *to chop, hew, cut down or cut out*. So it seems this is the more likely, although not as memorable or exciting, origin of the name.

The good news is that our skill at performing Caesarean sections has improved considerably. The first known successful operation, where the mother survived in Britain didn't occur until the early nineteenth century, and techniques have continued to improve dramatically.

What happens during a Caesarean?

Whether you're having a planned or elective Caesarean, or labour hasn't gone according to plan and you need an emergency operation, the procedure will usually be similar.

- The obstetrician will explain what is going to happen, talk you through any potential problems and ask you to sign your consent to the procedure.
- The upper bit of your pubic hair will be shaved or clipped away, so no hairs can affect the healing of the wound.
- You will be given some antacid medication to settle your stomach. This stops anything coming back up into your throat and is especially important if you're having an emergency section and may have eaten recently.

- A drip will be put into your arm, this can keep you hydrated, allow any intravenous medication to be given and allows for transfusion if there are any problems.
- An anaesthetist will give you a regional anaesthetic. It will numb your pelvis and legs, but you'll stay awake. You should feel no pain during the operation, although you may feel a little rummaging around. I always say it feels like someone is doing the washing up in your tummy! Occasionally, with an emergency Caesarean, you might need a general anaesthetic, so you will be asleep for the birth.
- When you are numb, a tube will be put in to drain your bladder. This means you won't have to wee for yourself until you're back on your feet.
- Your lower body will be covered with sterile sheets and a screen will be put up so you can't see any of the surgical procedure.
- The surgeon will make a small cut two finger widths above the pubic bone, so it should be hidden under your bikini line.
- There will be a further cut into the womb and your beautiful baby will be lifted out into the world. Congratulations, you are a mum!
- The placenta is removed and you'll be neatly stitched back up, in layers. The scar should heal well, leaving a fine line that will be hidden by your knickers or swimwear. The whole procedure takes around an hour, and so long as you're not having a general anaesthetic, your birth partner should be able to stay with you to share the joy.

Dr Keith says:

When I perform a Caesarean section, I prefer to use the technique named the Joel-Cohen incision. This is where the skin is incised a small amount, and the tissues are stretched and manipulated to allow the effective delivery of the baby. None of the muscles are cut, and because the incisions are kept to a minimum, and the tissue is stretched instead, the tissues quickly contract to their normal positions. I advocate closure of the subcutaneous fat layer to reduce the risk of wound haematoma and in my experience the use of non-absorbable subcuticular prolene for the skin appears to produce a superior cosmetic result.

One thing I would say is that the best piece of advice I received before having kids is that if something happens and you end up having to have a section expect there to be lots of people in the operating theatre! It's not that something is going wrong or that the baby is in danger, lots of people are needed: surgeon, doctor assisting, anaesthetist, anaesthetist assistant, midwife etc are there as standard. It is a busy room!

~ Lindsey, Kilkeel

Elective Caesarean section

My birth plan was to have an elective Caesarean section and the plan went without a hitch. I wanted a planned C-section because I wanted to control the outcome as much as possible in order to minimise the pain and trauma for myself and child. I find the idea of natural childbirth scary!

~ Johanna, London

Dr Keith says:

The Romans had a word for fear of childbirth: in Latin, it is tocophobia. That shows us it has been a common, and understandable, fear for at least two thousand years. It is absolutely normal to be nervous, especially if you are pregnant for the first time, or have had a difficult previous birth. My job, and the job of my fellow medical professionals is to help you understand what you can expect, so you aren't afraid of the unknown, and to work with you to manage both your rational and irrational fears.

An elective Caesarean section is planned before you go into labour. An operative delivery may be necessary because your baby is in an awkward position, like transverse or breech, because the placenta is low or because you are having twins or more.

Around one in ten women in the UK give birth by planned C-section. Most of these are for medical reasons, but the numbers are climbing because increasingly women are choosing an elective section. In a large study of breech births, babies who had an elective Caesarean did significantly better than those having a vaginal breech delivery, and so did their mums!

Your birth experience

With a planned Caesarean, there is more control over your birth experience, which may suit you and your birth partner. You will be able to mark a date in your diary when your baby will be born, so you can pack a bag, clear your partner's diary, fill the freezer and book a babysitter in advance.

If your baby is delivered by Caesarean section under regional anaesthesia, your partner will be able to sit with you in the operating theatre and share the joy and excitement of the birth. You should be able to bond with your baby immediately, with skin-to-skin contact.

I have found that an elective Caesarean is a positive way to enter the world, and you have the benefit of modern medications including antibiotics, and injections to stop blood clots, to prevent any problems.

Too posh to push?

This phrase was coined by newspapers to describe middle-class or successful women who choose a Caesarean because it fits in better with their life. One of the reasons people like the sound of an elective Caesarean is that it is a planned birth, so you know exactly when your baby is going to come, unlike vaginal birth babies who rarely turn up on time!

Gail Johnson, professional advisor for education and research at the Royal College of Midwives, said of Caesareans:

It's not a lifestyle choice, and although it's a safe operation, it does carry more risks than a vaginal birth.

It's a difficult conundrum and the debate rages on. The safest form of delivery would be an uncomplicated vaginal birth, and many women (over 50%) do manage to achieve this. But we have no truly accurate way of predicting who will have an uncomplicated vaginal birth. In my experience, and it's backed up by surveys, the women who are most dissatisfied with their birth experience are those who have an instrumental delivery or an emergency section.

Elective Caesareans would avoid these emergencies, but if we did a section on everyone to make it as safe as possible, we would be exposing many women to an unnecessary operation, which inevitably has complications which a straightforward vaginal birth doesn't. However, the complications associated with a planned Caesarean section are probably less than those of an instrumental delivery, and certainly less than those suffered by women who have major pelvic trauma following a vaginal birth.

I believe in giving women all the information available, so they can make an informed choice about planning the birth that is right for them.

Emergency Caesarean section

Sometimes birth doesn't go according to plan. It's a complex and delicate process which can need a helping hand. Maybe labour gets stuck and fails to progress, or your little one shows signs of distress, or your baby is breech and things are getting a little tricky, it can be safest for you and your baby to have a surgical birth.

An emergency section sounds frightening, and you may picture panic and running down corridors. But I'm glad to say that things are rarely that urgent. An emergency section usually describes an operation that has not been planned in advance.

This may not be the birth you described and intended in your birth plan, but the priority for everyone in the delivery room is that both you and your baby are healthy.

Your birth experience

Some women who have to have a Caesarean section feel a little cheated out of the childbirth experience, especially if it happened as an emergency.

> *A Caesarean is very scary and draining for the maternal body.*
>
> **~ Michelle, London**

Dr Keith says:

Around fifteen per cent of births in the UK are unplanned Caesarean sections, so it worth considering this as a potential outcome. The good news is that there is often time for you to have regional anaesthetic, so your partner can be present to share the experience and if there are no problems you should be able to have rapid skin-to-skin contact.

How many Caesarean sections are safe?

There's simply no easy answer to this question, we don't have a cut-off number of C-sections that can be considered safe. It really depends on the individual. One woman in the UK has had seven successful sections, with no problems, while others have had significant complications after their third.

Dr Keith says:

The first section will leave scars. This will make subsequent sections more difficult for your surgeon. The operation is likely to be longer and there is a small risk of damage to the bowel or bladder. On rare occasions, there have been reports of the baby being cut too.

Caesarean deliveries are at increased risk of:

Bleeding

There is a risk of bleeding after a Caesarean, but this increases with the number you have. Sometimes it's difficult to control heavy bleeding and there is a danger of needing a hysterectomy, or a womb removal, to stop life-threatening haemorrhage. In research, the risk of hysterectomy increased from less than one in a hundred (0.65%) after the first Caesarean to over one in forty (2.41%) after the fourth.

Placental problems

Repeat sections can increase the danger of the placenta growing into the scar, so it is abnormally attached to the womb wall. This can cause problems with the third stage of labour, retention of the placenta and sometimes severe haemorrhage and even the need for an emergency hysterectomy.

Because of this increasing level of danger, most obstetricians usually recommend that you limit your number of children to three. This is worth considering when you plan your first elective section.

Dr Keith says:

I've successfully delivered the babies of a number of patients who have had five or six Caesareans, but the risk definitely increases with increasing numbers such that I recommend careful family planning.

"One of the best ways to increase bonding is to encourage skin to skin contact."

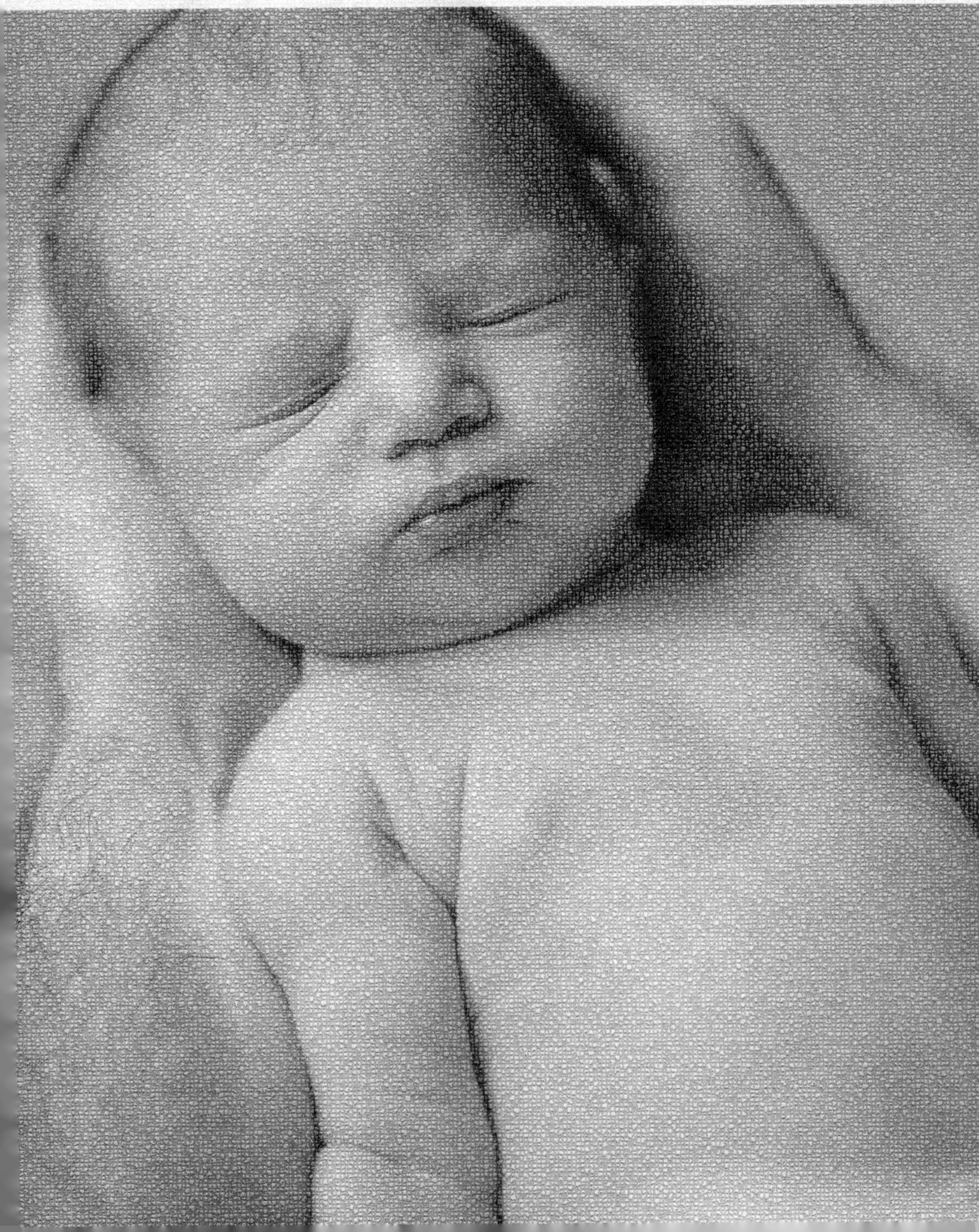

50

DOES EVERY MUM BOND WITH THEIR BABY?

Most mums expect to look at their baby and feel an instant magical sense of love and connection. It's true that some women look at the baby lying in their arms and feel an immediate emotional pull, but lots of women don't. Many mums take time to bond, not because they're bad mothers but because pain, problems in labour and the sheer exhaustion of the postnatal period can make it difficult.

It's really important not to worry or feel guilty if that's you. With time and support, the connection will come and there are some ways of helping the bonding process:

Skin-to-skin

One of the best ways of increasing bonding is to have early skin-to-skin contact.

When I help deliver babies, and I've had the honour and privilege of assisting with the beginning of thousands of little lives, I am a big believer in the importance of the early human touch.

The natural way

For me it's instinctive. I remember years ago when I was a student doctor, sometimes even perfectly healthy babies were whipped away from the mum, wiped, wrapped and returned some time later, perfect and packaged in a blanket. The sudden separation didn't seem right.

Your baby has been inside you for nine months; they've been surrounded by your warmth, your scent and the constant drum of your heart-beat. Being propelled into the cold, bright world must seem harsh and unsettling. By laying your little one straight on your body, against your skin with no fabric to separate the two of you, that special contact is being maintained. They'll be able to hear your heart, smell your skin and your body will radiate warmth and welcome. The touch of their skin will also stimulate your body to release the feel-good hormone oxytocin, which creates a feeling of calmness, closeness and attachment—it's a lot like falling in love.

Put simply, skin-to-skin contact is comforting for your baby, good for you and a wonderful way of establishing the bond between the two of you as separate human beings.

The sensitive time

I'm glad to say that the instinctive 'correctness' of skin-to-skin contact is backed up by medical evidence. Separation and swaddling can affect the interaction between mother and infant and make it more difficult to establish breast-feeding. It seems that there may be an early sensitive period after the birth, of up to two hours, during which close contact between mother and infant may have a positive impact on their relationship even a year later.

Safety first

Please don't get me wrong. The health of mother and baby has to come first. Skin-to-skin contact must never compromise the well-being of either. Post-natal bleeding or resuscitation of the infant has to be a priority. Sometimes it may be difficult for you to hold your baby straight after the birth, for example, if you've had a Caesarean or your baby needs special care. Try not to worry too much about this, your midwife or the paediatrician will help you have skin-to-skin contact as soon as it is safe to do so.

More and more neonatal units are now trying an exciting technique called kangaroo care. It's a way of caring for low-weight or preterm babies outside the incubator. It's about carrying your baby like a mummy kangaroo carries a baby joey, strapped to your bare chest so your body acts like a living incubator. Research seems to show that it may reduce rates of infection and hypothermia and may even decrease the length of hospital stay, so it's worth discussing with the hospital team.

I never felt that immediate bonding with my babies. I felt really bad because I was a paediatric nurse, I was used to looking after babies and I expected to feel that magical feeling when you look at your newborn. But I didn't I looked at them and thought 'that's a baby.' I never felt that connection, so I almost felt like I'd failed at the first hurdle.

I never told anyone how I felt because I thought it was bad, that it was something I should have felt.

The best thing for me was caring for the baby on a day-to-day basis and those feelings gradually fell into place. Now my children are the most important things in my life.

~ Your Pregnancy Doctor paediatric nurse Katie Hannant

If you're struggling to bond

Skin-to-skin contact will help at any time after the birth. Concentrate on the day-to-day care of your baby; cuddle, hold and feed them and with time the closeness will come. Baby massage can be brilliant at soothing a baby and improving bonding at the same time.

Above all, don't be afraid to share your worries and concerns. Many women feel the same, and your midwife, GP and health visitor will understand and offer support without judgment. Sometimes, bonding problems can be linked to emotional or mental distress for which you'll need expert help to begin the process of recovery:

Postnatal depression

Many women feel that the time after the birth with their beautiful new baby should be the happiest of their lives. But exhaustion, isolation, the stress of being responsible for a new life and the hormonal changes after the birth can mean that too often, it is anything but.

Mental illness affects around one in ten mothers in the postnatal period, but too often new mums feel ashamed about their emotions and struggle on with no treatment or help.

Breedagh Hughes from the Royal College of Midwives said that postnatal depression is still a taboo topic.

There is this societal expectation that when a woman gives birth she should be happy, jolly and delighted with herself. In fact, women who suffer from postnatal depression, try to compensate by trying to be a perfect mother, but emotionally there is nothing there.

Hopefully increased awareness, together with better access to therapy, medication and specialist mother and baby units will mean that women in need will get the help they need.

Do I have postnatal depression?

We all have good and bad days, and it's normal to feel irritable and tearful when you've been up all night with a crying infant. But women with postnatal depression will usually suffer from some, or all of the following symptoms, for many days over a period of at least two weeks.

- Persistent feeling of sadness; you may be tearful or you may feel flat and emotionless
- Loss of interest in the world and in things you used to enjoy
- Feeling tired and lacking in energy all the time
- Having difficulty bonding with your baby or feeling distant and detached
- Struggling to leave the house and avoiding contact with others
- Having difficulty concentrating, remembering things and making decisions
- Experiencing frightening and worrying thoughts; this could be about your abilities as a mother, ideas of suicide, or thoughts of hurting your baby

If you think you may be affected, it's important to get help as soon as possible. The sooner you act, the sooner you can get the help you need to feel better. With the right treatment and help, most women make a full recovery.

It can be hard to be reasonable and objective when you're feeling low. But try to remember that depression is a disease. It's not your fault and you didn't cause it. If you are having disturbing thoughts about your baby, that doesn't make you a bad person. The professionals are there to help you, and to keep you together with your baby while you get the therapy, medication and self-help guidance to help you recover from this difficult condition.

Baby blues

Very many women, around half of all new mums, feel tearful, emotional and upset during the first week after the birth. These, so-called baby blues are thought to be linked to the changes in hormone levels after giving birth. They should settle on their own by the time your baby is ten days old, rest whenever you can and accept any help offered.

If the feelings of sadness, exhaustion and anxiety don't settle, it may be more serious, so see your midwife, health visitor or doctor for some help and advice.

Getting help

Postnatal depression can be scary, lonely and difficult to deal, but you are not alone, effective treatments and support are available:

Self-help

Changing your diet, exercising regularly, getting enough rest and sharing with friends can help you deal with your feelings of depression.

Psychological therapies

There are many different talking treatments that can either be carried out individually or as part of a group session. Your doctor can talk through the options available in your area. These could include:

Cognitive behavioural therapy. CBT is a type of counselling that focuses on changing negative ways of thinking, it can help you deal with panic attacks, anxiety, stress and negative thinking.

Counselling. A counsellor can help you talk through your feelings, so you can understand and cope with them. If you find this process difficult, it can help to have antidepressants at the same time.

Support groups

Often, talking with other mums can help you understand that lots of other people are going through the same thing, so you can share tips, stories and support. Friends and family can be a huge help practically and emotionally but sometimes it can help to speak to someone from outside the family unit.

Medication

Medication can make a huge difference to your mental health, allowing you the space to heal. There are a number of effective anti-depressants that are safe to take during breastfeeding; talk to your GP about the pros and cons.

Coping with birth trauma

Sometimes despite the best planning and pregnancy care, birth doesn't go to plan. Childbirth can be painful, difficult and distressing and some women may suffer flashbacks, stress and ongoing problems after their experience. This can affect their wellbeing and their ability to bond with their baby.

What is post-traumatic stress disorder?

Post-traumatic stress disorder (PTSD) is our mind and body's natural reaction to a traumatic or frightening event. You may have heard the term used in the context of soldiers after combat, people who have experienced natural disasters or people who have been violently attacked or raped. But any scary or upsetting situation can lead to the symptoms of PTSD, and that can include childbirth. Labour can be frightening, and if there are signs of fetal distress, bleeding or emergency intervention, women may feel a loss of control and terror that their baby may suffer serious injury or die. This can predispose to birth trauma.

What are the symptoms?

PTSD is a group of symptoms experienced after a stressful experience. Women who are affected may feel extreme fear combined with a sense of utter helplessness. They may re-experience the event, with persistent flashbacks and intrusive and upsetting memories. These recollections will often trigger a visceral response, with feelings of anxiety, panic and fear resurfacing.

Because of the distress caused by the memories, most women affected will try to avoid thinking or talking about the birth, although some may go over and over the experience in an obsessive way. PTSD can cause much more than fear and anxiety, sufferers may struggle to sleep and concentrate and may feel angry, agitated or depressed.

Fight and flight

When you are dealing with birth trauma, it can seem as if you are going mad and that there is no way out. But I can only assure you that this is a normal human reaction to a challenging and traumatic time.

Your body's response to these flashbacks is totally instinctive and out of your control. It is part of your primitive fight-or-flight reflex, designed to help us face up to a physical challenge or safely escape. This was useful when we were cave-dwellers but can be less helpful when the source of stress is sustained and coming from your own memory.

PTSD is not about being weak-willed; it is something you cannot stop without professional help and support.

Who is likely to suffer PTSD?

This question isn't easy to answer. Yes, women who have experienced difficult births with interventions and problems with their baby can be at risk. Some distressing events would traumatise anyone. But often birth trauma can be a very personal thing. Cheryl Beck was quoted in Nursing Research as saying:

Birth trauma is in the eye of the beholder.

These words are absolutely true. It is the way that an individual woman experiences and understands the birth that is key. Loss of control, dignity and a lack of trust in staff can make birth trauma more likely.

Treatment of trauma

As an obstetrician, I strive to prevent PTSD developing by carefully managing the birth with excellent pain relief and intervention when necessary. However, prevention involves more than excellent technical care. Providing detailed information and explanation of any procedures, ensuring that consent is fully informed and making sure that at all times the mother and father are treated with dignity and respect can improve confidence, the feeling of control and wellbeing.

The impact of PTSD

Birth trauma can impact on relationships, bonding with your baby and your willingness to have another child, so it is essential to seek help. It is a separate condition from postnatal depression and needs a different approach, although the two can frequently co-exist. Antidepressants alone may not help; a talking therapy is usually necessary to help you overcome your distress.

Your first calling point should be your doctor or midwife to talk through your feelings. Some women find that going through the maternity notes, so each stage of labour can be explained and rationalised, really helps them start to come to terms with their experience. Your doctor can also refer you for counselling to help process your feelings, this may be in the form of cognitive behavioural therapy or psychotherapy.

You are not alone in this experience, as many as one in fifty mums can suffer ongoing birth trauma. There is help available so you can start to understand the difficulties of the birth and move forwards with the rest of your life.

With all your questions answered, it's now time for me to wish you a healthy pregnancy, a positive birth experience and a safe delivery. If you want to find out more about birth plans, pain relief and all of pregnancy's pitfalls there's an enormous amount of support and information available on **YourPregnancyDoctor.com**.

There is also expert advice about life with your new baby from our medical-led team of health professionals. Whether you're concerned about breast feeding, burping or baby poo, **YourPregnancyDoctor.com** has all the information you need to survive the first few weeks with your beautiful new baby.

97450649R00212

Made in the USA
Columbia, SC
17 June 2018